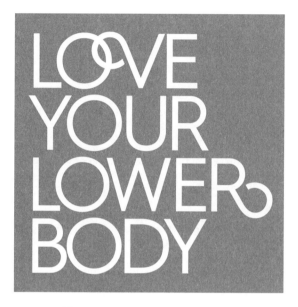

LOVE YOUR LOWER BODY

The 8-Week Plan to Sculpt a Slender, Strong, and Beautiful Physique

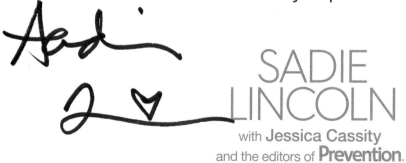

SADIE LINCOLN

with **Jessica Cassity**
and the editors of **Prevention**.

RODALE.

Prevention is a registered trademark of Rodale Inc.

Printed in the United States of America

Rodale Inc. makes every effort to use acid-free ⊗, recycled paper ♲.

Exercise photographs by Thomas McDonald/Rodale Images
Test panel photographs by Zach Shapiro
Before photographs provided by Annie Eeds and Robyn Conley Downs
Contents photograph by James Farrell

Book design by Carol Angstadt

Library of Congress Cataloging-in-Publication Data is on file with the publisher.

ISBN 978–1–62336–277–5 direct hardcover

2   4   6   8   10   9   7   5   3   direct hardcover

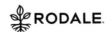

RODALE.

We inspire and enable people to improve their lives and the world around them.
For more of our products visit **prevention.com** or call 800-848-4735.

To my husband, Chris, and my children, Audrey and Drew, for reminding me that the in-between moments also make me healthy—like celebrating a loose tooth or a kiss good night.

Contents

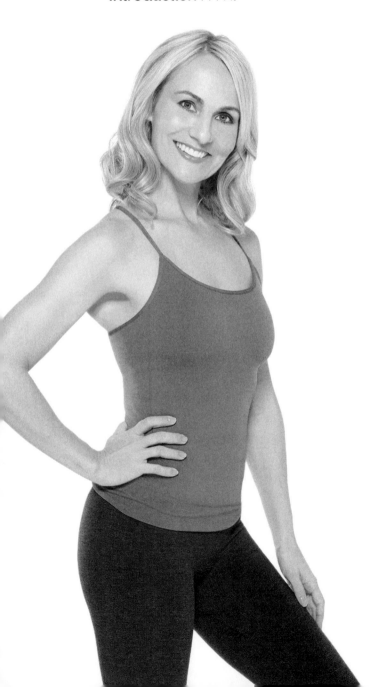

Foreword

AS FITNESS EDITOR FOR *PREVENTION* MAGAZINE, I'M ALWAYS LOOK-ing for new ways to help our readers achieve their health and fitness goals. Every workout that makes its way into our pages has to be doable, fun, and incredibly effective. It also has to energize you, inspire you, and make you feel and look like the best version of yourself.

Fitness expert Sadie Lincoln agrees, and her incredible fitness method, barre3, is built on the same principles. I met Sadie a few years ago, when barre classes were big and only getting bigger. I gravitated toward barre3 because I felt that Sadie's approach perfectly matched the *Prevention* fitness philosophy. Together we developed Love Your Lower Body, an amazing plan that provides phenomenal results. It utilizes the barre3 method, which combines the sculpting power of ballet barre work with elements of Pilates and yoga to transform and lift the entire body—especially the areas we all want to target, like the belly, butt, waist, hips, and thighs.

Sadie also understands what it takes to get in shape—and stay there—in your thirties, forties, and beyond. Which is why she partnered with physical therapists to develop moves that lessen back pain instead of aggravate it, and that you can easily modify to work with your individual needs and fitness level. She even divided her workouts into 10-minute segments so that anyone, no matter how busy, could squeeze them into their schedule.

Whether you've been looking for a fitness plan to help you get started, you want to maximize your results in minimum time, or you want to develop a beautiful figure and a healthful approach to eating and exercise, Love Your Lower Body is a plan that will help you achieve your goals.

Commit to the 10-minute workouts and clean eating tips, and watch your body, energy, and life transform. I promise that you'll be delighted with the results.

Jenna Bergen
Fitness Editor, **Prevention**

Acknowledgments

LOVE YOUR LOWER BODY IS BASED ON MY PERSONAL EXPERIENCE and expertise, but I couldn't have done it without my team of experts.

Deep gratitude goes out to my barre3 core team, including Amy Leclerc and Kait Hurley, who were my constant cheerleaders and support while simultaneously writing this book and running our dynamic and fast-growing company.

My talented team of barre3 master trainers helped me test this program, including Allison Beam, Catie Fahrner, Candace Ofcacek, Stephanie Rubenstein, Lisa Schale-Drake, and Heidi Waltermire.

Jennifer Curtiss-Thoman, ND, a talented nutritionist as well as a barre3 instructor, helped me assemble a team of our favorite chefs and nutrition mentors including Andrea Bemis, Abby Fammartino, Darcy Fix Harding, Jake Johnson, Katie Kahn, Viva Mertlich, and Stephanie Pearson, all of whom are aligned with our barre3 nutrition philosophy.

The plan wouldn't be what it is without the amazing test panelists who piloted the program and gave me invaluable feedback, especially: Audrie Abell, April Abernethy, Brooke Alley, Carie Behe, Cori Boynton, Jennifer Dashney-Longbine, Erin Dineen, Margueritte Kim, Jessica Klein, Sarah La Du, Frayn Masters, Zoe Murillo, Alex Nowlin, Christina Post, Megan Schendel, Angie Thomason, and Michelle Tubbs.

To my mom, Sonja Snyder: Thank you for helping me edit this book and for being a huge influence on my career as a fitness and wellness educator. I love you.

This book would not be in your hands if it weren't for my team at Rodale. Thank you to Marielle Messing, Carol Angstadt, Hope Clarke, Brooke Myers, Faith Hague, Jenna Bergen, and Bari Lieberman for embracing my vision and making this book a reality.

Last but certainly not least, I lucked out by getting to work with Jessica Cassity, a bright and talented writer who cares about this program as much as I do and was the perfect fit for this project: Not only is she a barre3 instructor, but she is also a former fitness editor for *Prevention* magazine.

Introduction

YOU MAY THINK YOU'RE READING A WORKOUT BOOK, BUT WHAT you're really holding in your hands is the key to whole-body health and a balanced life. That's a lot to promise on day 1 of our journey, but hear me out: This book isn't just a means to learn some new exercise moves. It is a way for you to discover how to live better and reach the goals you have for yourself, including weight loss, a toned body, reduced stress, and more energy. In opening up this copy of *Love Your Lower Body,* you are on the road to a whole new method of working out: one that is fun and easy to do anywhere; that leaves you feeling energized, not depleted; that adds joy to your day, not stress; and that still shrinks inches all over, particularly in those hard-to-tone trouble spots like your belly, hips, and thighs. You're also about to embark on a brand-new approach to food, one that nourishes your whole body and helps you shed extra weight.

What kind of workout can accomplish all that? Love Your Lower Body is an 8-week plan that is based on barre3, a fitness style I developed. It takes the standard ballet barre workout and blends in the influences of yoga, Pilates, and traditional fitness. You've probably heard of barre workouts, which are popping up all over the world, from metropolitan hubs like New York City to midwestern cities like St. Louis. Barre workouts are exciting because they quickly tone and shape your entire body. I love the fast changes I see in my clients' bodies, but what I love even more are the long-term transformations that happen. My signature barre3 program is more than a barre workout: It's a whole-body wellness and nutrition philosophy designed to give you the long, lean lines of a dancer and the power and strength of an athlete—all while helping you find a happier, more balanced mind-set. Thousands of clients love barre3 because it's fun to do and because it works.

Now I have teamed up with *Prevention* magazine to take the best of my barre3 studio workouts and nutrition program and create a plan just for you. You can do it at home or on the go. You don't need expensive gym equipment or much exercise space. And the nutrition program will satisfy even the pickiest eaters. All this plan requires is an open mind and a willingness to try.

Love Your Workout—Really!

I know you're excited to dive right into the Love Your Lower Body plan, but before you read on, take a moment to ask yourself why you bought this book. What is your objective? Is it to feel better about your body? To lose weight? To tone and shape your thighs? Or maybe to learn more about this barre craze you keep seeing everywhere? Whatever your reasons, I invite you to open your mind to some new ideas and find ways to make this plan your own.

My primary goal is to give you an exercise and diet program that you can integrate into your life so that exercise isn't a chore, but something you actually look forward to. The workouts in this book are designed to be done in small spaces (such as a galley kitchen or a small hotel room) and will take as few as 10 minutes a day. The recipes you'll discover in the nutrition portion of the book are simple, delicious, and based on a whole foods approach to eating. As you work your way through these meals and snacks, you'll learn a formula for healthy eating that you can use to make your favorite dishes even healthier.

My approach works, but don't just take my word for it: Throughout my more than 2 decades of experience as a fitness professional, I've witnessed thousands of success stories—including my own. Plus, we tested the Love Your Lower Body plan on more than 2 dozen women, and the results were astounding. They lost substantial pounds and inches within weeks of starting the program. Exercise and eating well became something they wanted to do, not only because of how it made them look but also because of how it made them feel: healthier, happier, and more energized. And the plan really is doable: All 27 participants successfully completed the 8-week program because it was fun and easy to follow. Each week, they were motivated by how fast their bodies were changing, but they were also inspired by the way this program improved their overall well-being. This is why I think of Love Your Lower Body as not only a diet and workout formula but a guide to whole-body health. You will certainly see some amazing transformations in the mirror, but the real rewards are on the inside.

WHERE ARE YOU NOW?

Pop quiz time! On a scale of 1 to 10, with 1 being "loathe it" and 10 being "love it," how would you rate your lower half? Don't overthink it. Just pick the number that best describes how you feel, right now, about your hips, thighs, and waistline. Got it? Commit this number to memory, or better yet write it down here: _____. In 8 weeks' time, ask yourself the same question again, and there's going to be a big change, not just in how you rate your looks but also in the way you see yourself. Even before this 8-week plan is finished, you will look in the mirror and really like what you see, particularly from the waist down. If you're like the two dozen women who tested this program, you'll also experience a host of other changes, from an improved attitude to better quality of sleep. As the workouts and eating choices become a natural part of your daily routine, you'll gain confidence that the life changes you've made will continue to transform your body and your habits long after the 8-week plan is over.

As the title suggests, one major goal of these workouts is to help you *love* your lower body. I'm going to guess that for many women, thinking of this region of your body conjures up emotions ranging from despair to hope. The trouble zones women worry about most all fall below the beltline. From belly fat to extra weight on the hips, butt, and thighs, these are the areas that plague us, the areas that almost any woman you ask will say she would like to strengthen, tone, and firm. I'm here to tell you that it is possible to start loving your lower half. My clients have watched their bodies become stronger and slimmer with small changes to their diet and daily activity. So hang on to hope and do away with despair. These next 8 weeks are going to be a period of new habits, self-discovery, and successes, small and large. I'm excited to be your guide on this journey.

Carry Your Curves with Confidence

Before we rework your body, let's talk attitude. Despite how you may feel about your body right now, curves are inherently good. For centuries, women with hourglass figures have symbolized health and fertility in artwork. And scientific studies (as well as locker room polling) reveal that curves are typically thought of as an asset. Most girls start to develop a rounder figure during puberty, when their bodies begin to naturally store fat in the breasts, belly, hips, and thighs. These curves may change size and shape with age, with weight gain or loss, and with pregnancy and motherhood, but in general, once you develop curves, they're here to stay—it's simply a part of womanhood. When I hear my friends complain about the size of their thighs, I remind them that those legs carry them around all day. Without that muscle mass, none of us would be able to do the things we love, like go hiking or play tag with our kids. I'm proud of my natural, feminine frame and all it can do, and I want you to be proud of your shape and your abilities, too. This plan isn't designed to give you an unnatural boyish shape or make you feel bad about your size—my goal is to give you the best body you can have, which, first and foremost, is a strong, shapely, and flexible one.

But—and you knew there had to be a "but" coming—carrying a lot of excess fat around those gorgeous curves can be harmful to your health. Statistically speaking, there's a high chance that you fall into this category: A staggering 69 percent of Americans are now considered overweight, according to the Centers for Disease Control and Prevention, and 36 percent of the population is obese. As a person's weight goes up, so do her health concerns. The National Institutes of Health warns that the higher your body mass index (also known as BMI, a measure of body fat calculated using your weight and height), the greater your risk of heart disease, high blood pressure, stroke, certain types of cancer, osteoarthritis, and sleep apnea, among other illnesses. There is such a strong association between obesity and type 2 diabetes that doctors and health journalists have coined the term "diabesity." These facts alone are alarming, but the news is worse when your excess weight is stored largely around your waistline: People who have significant fat stores around the belly—even if they are a relatively healthy weight—are twice as likely to die from any cause than people with skinnier middles, according to a study from the Mayo Clinic.[1]

Of course, the negative effects of excess weight aren't all physical. Being unhappy with your appearance can be a mental burden as well. I know what it's like to spend hours shopping for clothes that would cleverly disguise my body or even cropping photos so I was captured only from the waist up. This is an awful feeling—and one that many of us have experienced. I recently read that the average woman thinks dozens of negative thoughts about her body each day. I know how taxing that can be. There are so many things I'd rather have on my mind than my appearance, and I'm guessing you would, too. My hope for you is that as you get stronger and have more endurance, increased flexibility, and better balance, you'll start to appreciate your body more and be filled with confidence about everything you can accomplish.

My Fitness Odyssey

I love exercise. My passion for fitness started years ago, when I spent a lot of time in my living room with my mom, our Jane Fonda video, and a rad pair of leg warmers. My interest carried me all the way to UCLA, where I received my undergraduate degree in sociology while teaching any form of group exercise I could get trained in: high/low aerobics, step, slide, circuit, weight training, and kickboxing. It also led me to the College of William and Mary, where I earned my master's degree in education and accepted a graduate assistantship to develop the school's group exercise program. Not surprisingly, all of this led to a career in fitness: Right after grad school, I landed a job at 24 Hour Fitness, where I worked for 10 years. I helped develop the national group exercise program and, as part of the executive team, built the company brand to be one of the largest health clubs on the globe.

Ironically, while I was at 24 Hour Fitness, I rarely worked out at the gym. In my early twenties, while still a student, high-energy, high-intensity types of exercise were a good fit for my life and goals. I felt strong and had plenty of time to spend exercising. But as I got a little older, life changed dramatically. I worked in an office, which left me zapped at the end of the day. I got married, which meant I had to choose between spending time at the gym or spending time with my husband, Chris. And I experienced that dreaded metabolism slowdown so many of my clients had complained about. My body changed in ways I wasn't all that happy about, and the workouts I used to do left me feeling tired and depleted. I needed something completely different—something that fit into my life and that energized me to tackle the rest of my day.

So I tried yoga. This was a transformative experience, inside and out. For the first time in my life, I slowed down and listened to what my body really needed. I learned to move with intention and found power in resting some days and working hard on others, all based on how I felt. I learned to be less attached to an outcome such as how many calories I was burning or how hard my abs were. Instead, I focused deeply on how I was feeling in the moment. As soon as this shift happened, the extra weight I'd been carrying melted off. My energy skyrocketed. I felt more in touch with my body, my thoughts, and my moods than ever before. I was going to class several times a week and found that I actually walked out ready to be a better employee, friend, and wife. But then another change came: I had children. Suddenly, fitting in a 90-minute workout wasn't so easy, and toning my tush and abs was even harder. I loved the feel of yoga, the idea of balancing effort and ease, but my body was ready to move on to something new.

At this point, I'd tried just about every type of exercise out there. Yoga was too much of a time commitment. Pilates was expensive, and I found the equipment intimidating. Traditional fitness programs felt too masculine and competitive. The barre workouts I'd tried came close—but they triggered my lower-back pain, and I missed the warm, accessible culture of yoga. I was on a fitness odyssey, and it was about to lead me into uncharted territory.

All About barre3

When I set out to develop barre3, I wanted to create a fitness system that was accessible, fun, and highly efficient—a technique that included all of the things I love about exercise. I also wanted to forge a business model that supported the values my husband and I left our big corporate jobs for. We built barre3 around our desire to make work a balanced lifestyle. So I pulled in my know-how about traditional fitness programs and brought in the wisdom of yoga, the grace of using the ballet barre, and the strength of functional training techniques such as Pilates. My goal was to create a one-stop fitness style that delivered all of the physical and mental benefits you would expect from these various forms of exercise. I wanted to build in the calorie burn of moderate aerobic activity and the toning benefits of strength training. I wanted to highlight the important muscles of the core and help people realize that concentrating on your moves and your breath can help you calm your mind. Most important, I wanted a workout that felt good during the sessions and even better after.

Today, with more than 50 studios around the world and a following of my online workouts and nutrition programs in more than 60 countries, I am extremely confident that barre3 works. Each week, I receive dozens of messages from people who have had success with our workouts. I hear from women who finally shed stubborn baby weight, mother-daughter duos who attend classes together week after week, and people who have used barre3 to rebound from injuries. But the people I hear from the most are the ones who are achieving results with barre3 that they haven't been able to get from other workouts.

I will be the first to admit that the benefits barre3 delivers aren't completely unique. Indoor cycling classes burn a tremendous number of calories, kettlebell workouts can build major muscle, and yoga can stretch your body and relax your mind. What's different about barre3, and the reason it has such a passionate following, is that it feels easier to do than a lot of other workouts. It combines the best parts of a number of different types of training, which means it's ultra-efficient. Because barre3 uses small movements, it's easy to work this way of exercising into your life, doing moves all day long if you want. Also, barre3 focuses on the whole body—including what you eat.

The barre3 nutrition formula is based on a collective wisdom gained from my upbringing on whole foods and the latest research on how food functions in the body. My team of experts includes weight-loss professionals, scientists, functional nutritionists, doctors, and chefs who specialize in simple healthy recipes. They ensure that the foods I recommend taste great and give your body the fuel it needs.

One of my clients, Annie Eeds, who has lost more than 75 pounds over 18 months, had this to say about barre3:

> I spent years trying various exercise routines, but nothing worked: Gym classes left me exhausted, running caused me joint pain, and working out with a personal trainer lightened my wallet, if not my body. I gave popular diets a shot, too, but even though I counted calories and points and probably drank my weight in powdery shakes, my waist kept ballooning while my health declined. Then I discovered barre3. The moves felt like they were shaping my body from the inside out, but without pain or buckets of sweat. The focus on control and form and "making it my own" helped energize my mind, body, and soul. The barre3 food philosophy helped me understand how to make well-balanced meals that fuel my body and brain throughout the day. I truly have finally found my dream program, and it has changed the course of my future. I have steadily lost weight, gained confidence, changed my body, formed friendships, and inspired others. Thanks to barre3, I feel like I got my life back.

The Love Your Lower Body program is designed to balance ease and effort, to help you change your body without having to completely change your life. I can't wait to share my plan with you and to help you feel and be at your best. Welcome to the program—let's get started!

Chapter 1

Get Ready to LOVE Your LOWER BODY

PICTURE YOURSELF STANDING TALL, HEAD HELD HIGH, CHEST OPEN, and abs drawn in (tight). You step back into a lunge, hold this position for a moment, then you start to move, lifting and lowering your hips in just 1-inch movements. At first, it might feel easy. There's no impact on your joints, and the movements are small and controlled. To someone who's walking by, it might not even look like you're moving. But after just a few reps, your lower body starts to heat up. Your glutes—the muscles in your seat—are fully contracted with no chance to rest. Your quads—the muscles at the fronts of your thighs—are firing at full capacity. Your hamstrings—those often-neglected muscles at the backs of your thighs—are quickly reaching fatigue. You're barely moving, but your body is clearly burning fat and building muscle. This combination of little effort for lots of effect is the barre3 secret and the foundation of the Love Your Lower Body program.

The 8-week Love Your Lower Body plan is proven to get results—just ask the 27 women who tested it while we were writing the book. Angie Thomason ended the program stronger and more flexible than ever, and her toned and smaller body made her feel sexy. Frayn Masters's shape transformed, giving her legs more definition and shrinking her belly by almost 4 inches! Erin Dineen, who lost 15 pounds and more than 11 inches, felt firmer all over and had an easier time doing her favorite sports. Week after week, these women's bodies were changing, even though they were exercising for only 10 minutes at a time. They had lithe legs, shapely seats, and whittled-down waistlines. Women like April Abernethy, who lost 7 pounds in just 7 days on the program, were astounded by their results, but I wasn't. I've known for years that this type of exercise really works. That's why I'm so happy to share Love Your Lower Body with you.

Finding Balance

What makes Love Your Lower Body different is the ease of this program. The workouts fit around your obligations rather than interrupting them. The moves train multiple trouble zones at once, which allows you to spend less time exercising and more time enjoying the other parts of your day.

The snacks and meals keep your energy strong and steady all day long—no spikes and crashes. My goal isn't only to make you look and feel better, it's to bring balance to your life.

Balance is the key to success on this plan, and really to anything you do. This isn't simply my opinion—it's probably something you've already experienced, particularly in the weight-loss realm. If you don't have some give along with the take, you'll quickly burn yourself out and be right back where you started. This was one of the biggest lessons I learned during my own fitness journey and one I impart to all of my clients, including you.

The truth is, the most effective workout isn't necessarily the one that pro athletes or celebrities follow or the one that produces the most sweat. The most effective workout is the one that you actually commit to, despite the length of your to-do list or the sleepless night you just suffered through or the holiday trip you have planned. My goal in creating this plan was to make the meals tasty and satisfying and the workouts fun and simple enough that you start craving them to break up midafternoon boredom, to give you an extra surge of early-morning energy, or to help you shrug off stress at the end of a long day. I want this to be a program you want to do, and if you ask the Love Your Lower Body test panelists: Mission accomplished. Here's what Jennifer Dashney-Longbine had to say: "As someone who has never been particularly fit, even when I was thin, it's truly a miracle that I now look forward to working out. For years, I've heard women talk about wanting to work out, but I just couldn't relate. Now I feel the same way—I actually want to fit in exercise! What a change!"

Small Commitment, Big Change

For the next 8 weeks—and hopefully beyond—you'll follow the Love Your Lower Body workout formula, which firms and tones, burning fat and calories without any huffing and puffing. With each move, you'll experience the grace of ballet with the wisdom of yoga and the strength of Pilates, all without any fancy choreography. You'll build muscle without bulk, elevate your heart rate and burn calories with ease, and increase your flexibility. You'll eat a balanced diet of delicious meals so satisfying that you'll break free from some of the unhealthy foods you crave. I live this plan. I have been following this diet for years and have seen these moves work on my body and thousands of others. I developed this plan based on my own needs, and I am confident it will satisfy your needs, too.

The payoffs of this program are big, but the commitment is small. On some days, you may only need to do 10 minutes of activity (and the most you'll ever see on the schedule is 40 minutes). This workout is *that* effective at burning fat and strengthening the muscles in your hips, legs, and waistline. When it's time to eat, you can flip to one of my easy-to-prepare recipes, follow my suggestions for turning leftovers into a new dish, or simply reach for one of the grab-and-go snacks.

The benefits of the program may start with the workouts and meals, but they don't end there. With this book, you're going to learn how to be healthy all day long. The exercises and recipes are designed to make you live your whole life better, whether that means sitting at your desk with improved posture, having an easier time getting down to play with your babies or grandbabies, or beating your best time in a 5-K.

Many of the 27 women who initially tested Love Your Lower Body found that the self-focus I encourage—checking in with your body to see how the moves feel—helped them make better decisions in other areas of their lives, too. Some of these women reported that jump-starting their bodies with activity inspired them to spend less time sitting. Others gave up unhealthy habits like adding Splenda or salt to every meal. All reported feeling better about their bodies and themselves.

As you progress through the plan, don't be surprised if you experience the snowballing of positive change, with one good behavior leading to another. Scientists call this self-efficacy. Basically, when you make one healthy choice, your confidence gets a boost and you're more inclined to make another healthy choice. According to health researchers, women who start an exercise plan often begin to naturally make healthier food choices. If you picked up this book primarily for the workout, you may be pleasantly surprised that the diet portion of the Love Your Lower Body plan is just what you're looking for.

Perhaps you're worried that making so much change at once will be hard to stick with, but don't fret. A recent study from Stanford University's School of Medicine found that people who kicked off diet and exercise plans concurrently had better success than those who started with either a diet or workout plan and then tried to add more healthy behaviors later.[1] Scientists suspect that it might be easier, psychologically, to make one big change rather than a few medium-size changes. So I encourage you to embrace both the workouts and the nutrition components from the very beginning to get the most out of these next 8 weeks.

A Sneak Peek

The moves in this program range from ballet-inspired pliés to yogalike lunges to Pilates-based core blasters to signature barre3 moves designed by me and my team of experts. All work multiple muscles at once, so you're never challenging just one body part—and this cuts down on the overall time it takes to tone your entire body. I specifically selected the exercises in the book because they're incredibly effective and easy to learn. During Week 1, you'll do the 10 Transformative Minutes and the Standing Stretch. This two-part workout is the cornerstone of the entire program and is made of my favorite moves for lifting, shaping, and trimming the lower body.

From there, you'll learn new workouts each week, expanding your knowledge and deepening your practice for optimal results. My goal is to make sure you are never bored and are always challenged so that you don't plateau. In less time than you think, you'll gain stamina and strength and be able to hold poses for longer, get deeper into each position, and push your body to its edge—that muscle-shaking place where change happens. (You'll read more about these shaky-quakey "barre3 earthquakes" in Chapter 5!) That's why the program keeps working week after week: I give you options for each pose so you can discover how to increase or decrease the intensity depending on how you feel each day.

All the routines are gentle on the joints and effective at training the muscles and burning major calories. You may sweat a little, but these workouts are designed to feel less like an epic run on a treadmill and more like a deeply attuned yoga session. The movements are precise. I carefully set up each posture and then describe in detail how to get the most out of the exercise. I encourage you to take the time to read the instructions and then put the principles into practice by exploring each posture at your own pace. This process of reading and then doing will allow you to learn the moves and make them your own.

Every single test panelist I spoke with about the workouts discovered that over time, even the most basic exercises became more challenging and rewarding thanks to tiny adjustments in how they used their muscles and where they placed their weight. They learned how to modify the moves to have better form and alignment in their bodies, or to increase the intensity when they were ready for a new challenge. Over time, as you master each exercise, you will learn how to get the very most out of it. This program is designed to challenge and transform your body so you use it at its maximum potential.

I encourage you to try the workouts throughout the day, whether you're wearing fitness apparel, pajamas, or work clothes. Because the moves don't require any special equipment except, at times, a stable surface to hold on to (such as a countertop), you can fit in exercise while at your office, in your kitchen, at the playground, or after a run. In fact, some movements are so subtle you could even do them while standing in line at the store and no one would know!

Tone in 10 Minutes

All of this contributes to the success of the Love Your Lower Body workout, but it's the actual exercise schedule that has me most excited about this plan, and I know you'll appreciate it, too. The usual fitness programs are typically done in 30- to 60-minute blocks, but I know as well as anyone that it can be hard to set aside a full hour—or even a continuous 30 minutes—for fitness. If my kids aren't waiting for dinner, then I'm probably running late for a meeting. I get that you're busy—I'm busy, too. We all are. Lack of time is one of the main reasons people say they don't exercise. According to the U.S. Department of Labor, the average American woman spends just 13 minutes of each day exercising, which isn't a lot to work with. But it might be enough, at least some days.

A couple of years ago, my friend Amy called me to tell me that she had taken some of her favorite lower-body exercises from my longer classes and started to do them in short bursts throughout the day. At that point in her life, she had a newborn and a toddler at home and was strapped for time. She told me she wasn't going to let the fact that a long workout wasn't possible get in the way of a "great butt." So while stirring oatmeal, talking on the phone, and even nursing, she was doing barre3 pliés and leg lifts. And you know what? It really worked for her. Amy's story inspired me to develop short workouts that weave right into your packed schedule.

I started choreographing 10-minute workouts for this plan, which is just enough time to make your body feel the healthy effects of exercise, but not so much time that it becomes daunting to fit in. Over the next 8 weeks, you'll learn five of these 10-minute routines—and some special 5-minute routines as well. Some days, you'll do just one 10-minute sequence—your 10 Trans-formative Minutes—and other days, you'll include up to 40 minutes of work-outs of your choice, which you can do all at once or by spacing the short blocks of fitness around meals, during slow periods at the office, or while waiting for dinner to come out of the oven. A 40-minute workout might sound impossible to fit into your schedule, but four 10-minute sessions are easy to slip in. All day long, you'll be literally transforming your body, 10 minutes at a time, without feeling like you're giving up anything.

I love how simple these short fitness blasts are to squeeze in between appointments, but 10 minutes of exercise isn't a gimmick. Dozens of recent scientific studies show that shorter workouts may actually provide greater health benefits than longer ones. Regular 10-minute bursts of fitness can lower blood pressure and help regulate blood sugar more effectively than a longer workout—and they may burn more calories, too, thanks to the after-burn you get after each short session. As a built-in bonus, a few well-timed rounds will break up bouts of sitting, which can be extremely hazardous for your health. I'll share more on the benefits of short exercise sessions in Chap-ter 2, but know that the plan is designed to make your workouts more manageable, more convenient, more effective, and more fun. I've really enjoyed shifting to this new, flexible format, and I think you're going to like it, too.

DIY Workouts for a Plan That's Truly Yours

Each exercise is easy to learn yet challenging to do. I set up each position clearly then ask you to move slowly and with control so there's little chance for injury yet plenty of opportunity for you to get deep, really tapping the strength of your core, legs, and butt and even your back, arms, and shoulders. The movement sequences I created for this plan are designed to leave you feeling energized, not out of steam. The routines are easy enough to learn that you'll soon be able to do them anywhere, book in hand or not. I've included variations and modifications for exercisers of all abilities. My hope is that you'll find ways to make the movements work for you—modifying poses so they feel best on your body and fitting in exercise at the times of day that benefit your mind and muscles the most.

With Love Your Lower Body, there's no rigid schedule to follow. I suggest which exercise routines and how many minutes of exercise you should aim to fit in each week, and you decide which days will be your "long" days and whether to group your workouts into one routine or break them up throughout the day. This flexibility is meant to help you: If life's little surprises leave time for just one 10-minute workout on Monday, you can plan to set aside more time on Tuesday—or Wednesday. I've found that relieving the pressure of a rigid schedule is empowering. My goal is to give you the tools to make this an integrated way of life that feels authentic to who you are.

Good Eats: Hearty, Whole, and Healthful

This lifestyle philosophy also applies to the meal plan in this book. After all, there's more to loving your body than simply remembering to move it! You also need to be thoughtful about how you fuel your efforts. That's why

I've included more than 50 recipes for you to try, along with suggestions to help please every palate and satisfy dietary restrictions.

My entire barre3 team is passionate about good food. It's one of the things that bond us. On a given day, you might find bowls of almonds and berries in the conference room, healthy salads in the fridge, and green tea in about a dozen steaming mugs. We all eat healthfully, but we *never* count calories, and we never feel deprived. We celebrate whole foods, and in doing so, we crowd out unhealthy eating options.

I based the Love Your Lower Body eating plan on my personal food philosophy. The formula is quite simple: I eat whole foods, and I eat a balance of protein, healthy fats, and fiber in each and every meal. On a basic level, whole foods are easier for our bodies to digest, and they almost always contain more nutrients than processed foods. Many whole foods are also naturally balanced sources of nutrition. Take nuts, for example: They are essentially little prepacked balls of healthy fats, fiber, and protein, all of which are vital for keeping the body running at its peak. This is just one example of several key foods that will help you feel great on this plan.

While I refer to the eating philosophy of this plan as a "diet," I'm only using that word for the sake of simplicity. This isn't a typical diet. You'll feel full after meals, and you'll like the taste of the food. There's no need to buy a kitchen scale or plug the bites you've taken into a high-tech calorie-tracking site. The recipes take 30 minutes or fewer to prepare. To save even more time, I help you repurpose leftovers into delicious new meals for lunches or snacks.

Created with the help of chefs and nutritionists from my barre3 team, these delicious and easy meals will nourish your body and your taste buds. My instructors, clients, and the Love Your Lower Body test panelists tried them all and gave them rave reviews. Some of the women who tested the recipes were worried they would miss their comfort foods, things like cookies and french fries. But after less than a week without soda, coffee, breads, and salty processed foods, their sugar and salt cravings practically vanished, a true testament to the body's ability to recalibrate with the help of a healthy diet. When one tester admitted to popping open a diet soda midway through the program, she said she was surprised by the overly sweetened chemical taste. That experience was enough to make her swear off diet soda for good.

Some of the group's favorite recipes included the Chicken Tacos (page 253), the dessertlike Protein Power "Barre" (page 282), and the easy DIY Smoothie (page 226), DIY Muesli (page 232), and DIY Salad (page 240). This book includes only the recipes that also scored high with kids and spouses.

In addition to specific food suggestions, I'll give you the tools to help you determine whether your own favorite meals fit this new way of eating. If not, you'll learn how to alter them so they contain a healthy balance of protein, fat, and fiber. My hope is that the longer you follow this style of eating, the more you will experiment with new foods, flavors, and cooking styles and expand your recipe collection far beyond what you find in this book.

A Whole-Body Plan to Fit Your Whole Life

Scientists have spent years researching what makes a person commit to a weight-loss program, and the results are straightforward. People will follow a plan that's enjoyable, easy to do, and effective. That's it, and that's the secret to this workout. The reason the 27 panelists who tested it had so much success—and the reason you will, too—is that the Love Your Lower Body routine fits seamlessly into your life so that the payoff comes quickly.

It sounds pretty simple, right? If you were feeling intimidated about trying this program, I hope that reading this preview of the next 8 weeks eases your fears. The Love Your Lower Body plan is designed to be something you can start to follow the moment you pick it up, without a lot of extra planning. You may buy a few new ingredients at the grocery store— like quinoa or sunflower seed butter (which is my favorite)—but you don't need to invest in any new fitness gear, gadgets, or apparel (except, if you'd like, a core ball, which you can learn more about in the sidebar "Tools to Try" on page 85). On a typical day, you'll fit in a short block of exercise here and a healthy meal or snack there. And between it all, you'll manage the rest of your life—errands, deadlines, and, most important, spending time doing what you love to do. This plan is all about working smarter, not harder, and I'm not just talking about the moves. This sense of ease is something I hope you'll soon be able to apply to your entire life.

Over the next several chapters, you'll learn all about the science and about the diet and exercises in detail. But before we get into the nitty-gritty, let me answer a few questions I'm sure you're already forming.

Love Your Lower Body: Q&A

Q Why 8 weeks?

A In my experience, somewhere between 6 and 8 weeks of trying on a new lifestyle is enough to make it not only habitual but also preferable. On the Love Your Lower Body plan, 8 weeks is enough time for your cravings for unhealthy food to be replaced by cravings for foods that benefit you. It's also enough time for your body to start to crave exercise, even on your rest days. I created this program to help you learn to live a more fulfilling life, today and in the future. You may not know it now, but if you're anything like the other women who have tried this program, you'll wake up that first morning of Week 9 and reach for the same foods you've been eating and do the same exercises you've been doing throughout the program. This routine will no longer feel like the Love Your Lower Body plan—it'll just feel like life, and a good life at that.

Q What if I haven't worked out in years?

A I'll be the first to admit that exercise can be intimidating. To this day, I'm shy about walking into a new studio and trying something different. Will I look foolish? Will I be comfortable modifying the workout if certain exercises don't feel good? This fear hasn't gone away, even after my 20 years as a fitness professional. It's hard to try something new, to accept that it may take a little time to truly get "good." If you're feeling a tinge of this worry, it's natural. But in this case, it's also unnecessary. The beauty of working out with this book as your guide is that you can do the movements on your terms, and in private. I invite you to follow this program word for word or to move at your own pace, gradually getting comfortable with each stage of exercise on your own schedule. No one will judge you, no one will see if you accidentally lose your balance or if you take what feels like a lot of breaks. So don't judge yourself. Be proud of the effort you put into this and shrug off any missteps along the way.

The workouts in the coming chapters are clearly detailed, but be sure to read through all of the options to pinpoint the best workout for your body. I designed this plan so you can make it your own. I offer many modifications because every body is so different. The goal is to find grace in each posture while challenging yourself. Try the different options and see which feel best. Modifications can increase or decrease the intensity of an exercise, and they are included to help you find the best fit for your individual needs. Each of these moves is designed to give you the amazing results I know you want, including a toned body and more energy.

 ## Will I have to give up my favorite foods?

 This isn't a diet. It's a lifestyle change. I am going to ask you to give up some foods, but they are being omitted for good reasons. In this plan, we emphasize eating whole foods—things like leafy greens, whole grains, healthy fats, and lean proteins. These foods provide your body with the fuel, vitamins, and nutrients you need. Processed foods, which often contain all sorts of unnatural ingredients, are out because they are hard to digest and they change your body chemistry in a negative way. This program limits alcohol, coffee, and refined sugar because they contribute to increased blood sugar and fat stores. The protein gluten—which is found in several types of grains and therefore in foods like breads, cakes, and cereals—causes inflammation and blocks the absorption of essential nutrients, so it's also on the avoid list. But that's it. You're essentially eliminating a

small subset of all the food available. You still have hundreds of foods to choose from. If you're worried that you won't know what to do without these old staples, fear not: In addition to explaining my nutrition philosophy in greater detail in Chapter 3, I've also included dozens of recipes in Chapter 7 to help you learn how to put this style of eating to the test.

Q Does it really work?

A I've received rave reviews from thousands of satisfied barre3 participants, many of whom have been able to eliminate diabetes medications, recover from chronic pain, drop as many as four dress sizes, and even wear a bikini with confidence. But these clients were taking my 60-minute live studio classes or following my barre3 online workouts. It wasn't until 2012, when I wrote an article for *Prevention* magazine called "Ballet Boot Camp," that I realized I could help people by writing about my workouts. That program, which was a 30-day barre3 exercise and nutrition program, inspired amazing successes. I continue to hear from people who jump-started their weight loss with that plan and are still sticking to it. That experience made me want to do something more, something bigger. So I decided to write this book.

To be sure this brand-new plan really worked, my team introduced the program to 27 women and tracked their progress over the 8-week test period, charting weight, body fat, and inches lost, as well as muscle gained. We also measured things beyond the numbers, including body image, self-esteem, and energy levels. As the women tried each of the workouts and recipes, they helped us create the clearest, easiest-to-follow, and most effective plan. Their investment of time and effort really paid off: Almost immediately, people started to notice changes on the scale, in how their waistbands fit, in the muscle definition in their legs, as well as in the seat of their pants. By the end of the first week, some women had lost as many as 7 pounds; after 8 weeks, our top loser had dropped more than 18 pounds. But the results I am most proud of go beyond the scale. The vast majority of these women described the workouts as being fun and empowering them to feel good about their bodies. Many of the participants were amazed that they could eat delicious, satisfying food and do a workout that didn't exhaust them while getting the same results as a much stricter and more challenging program.

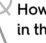 **How much time do I need to invest each day in this program?**

I've designed this program to fit into your life. Each workout is just 10 minutes. Some days you'll do one workout, other days you'll do three or four of these mini–fitness sessions. Once a week, you'll get a full day of rest. My goal is to make it easy to do these workouts all day long. Many women from the test panel were surprised how this approach made them *crave* exercise. The 10-minute workouts gave them more energy rather than leaving them exhausted. These short workouts will fit in between the things on your to-do list. You can work out while watching your kids play soccer, while stuck in your office on a conference call, or while waiting for a pot of water to boil. I keep food prep simple, too. The recipes are designed to be prepared in under 30 minutes, and I've included some of my favorite on-the-go options, which take no time at all. My hope is that this program doesn't make you feel like you're losing time in your day but that you are actually more efficient.

 What if there's no ballet barre in my house?

Full disclosure: I haven't installed a ballet barre at my house either, and for good reason. There are all sorts of things that can stand in for a ballet barre. After all, the main requirement is that you find a stable surface at waist height. Once you start looking around, you'll find all sorts of items that fit the bill. Some of my favorites are my kitchen counters, my dining room chairs, and the backs of the park benches near my kids' favorite playground. Certain moves do require a steadier surface than others. For instance, during Push-Pulls, you'll want to use your body weight to really press against the barre-like surface, so you'll be better off using a secure counter rather than a chair.

Q Can I follow this diet if I have food restrictions?

A Absolutely. With so many recipes to choose from, there are undoubtedly lots of options for everyone, from vegetarians to people with food allergies to the pickiest of eaters. And once you learn to follow this style of eating, you can begin to create your own meals and snacks that might better suit your tastes, preferences, and restrictions.

Q Can I do this workout even if I have an injury?

A As with all new exercise programs, if you have any concerns about getting started, you should consult your physician first. Most exercises are easy to modify, and I've included instructions to help you find a variation that feels best on your body. For example, if your knees are achy on all fours, I offer an option to do the exercise standing. However, if you have either a short-term or a chronic injury, or if you have any other concerns about exercise, I suggest you seek the professional opinion of your doctor before embarking on this journey.

Q Why is this workout plan going to work for me when so many others have failed?

A Think back to the reasons other exercise and nutrition plans didn't stick. It might be because of something wholly outside of your control, like suffering from an injury. But more likely, you let go of past attempts to exercise because it felt like a chore and a lot of work. You were probably constantly at the gym, or counting calories, or both. The program most likely felt like something that other "fit" people do—and not something that felt natural to you.

On the Love Your Lower Body plan, the idea is to work smarter, not harder. You won't ever need to block out a large chunk of time for exercise—just 10 minutes at a time. You don't need an exercise room. You can do this workout just about anywhere. You don't need

HOW WE TESTED THE PLAN

When my team reached Jessica Klein on the phone, you would have thought we had told her she had won the lottery—she was that happy. But for the 40-year-old mother of two and small business owner, being invited to test my 8-week fitness and diet plan felt like hitting the jackpot. "I couldn't believe I was picked," says Klein. "I was literally crying tears of joy."

This was a common response from the women we selected to test-drive the Love Your Lower Body workout and diet plan. Most were ready for a change and thrilled to be given the opportunity. These were women who had maybe heard about barre3 but who had been too intimidated—or too busy—to come to class. With this program, class came to them!

We kicked off the 8-week plan with a party of sorts—a get-together where they were introduced to the program. At the same time, we took their measurements, including weight, percentage of body fat, and inches around various spots (waist, hips, thighs, etc.), as well as things like mood, self-esteem, and energy level. Every 2 weeks, we checked in with the testers, updating their numbers. Seeing these changes helped keep the panelists motivated. On weeks when the number on the scale plummeted, they were overjoyed. On weeks when the scale didn't move as much, they were amazed to see how much their inches were still changing and how their moods and energy had improved.

These women made Love Your Lower Body come alive for me. They helped me work out the kinks in the workouts, perfect the recipes, and create a healthy whole-body program that really works, and for that I am truly grateful. These women also provided a lot of support and motivation for one another, sharing successes as well as the occasional frustration, and I know that this togetherness improved their results. Research shows that fitness buddies can drive change, so I encourage you to recruit a friend or two to harness this powerful energy that comes from a group of people making healthy shifts.

fancy workout attire (I often do these workouts in street clothes, and so can you). There will be no kitchen scales or strict portions on the diet plan. Instead, you'll try some delicious recipes, learn our simple eating principles, and set out on your own. Other plans set up barriers; this one takes them down.

Q How do you actually learn a workout from a book?

A At first, I was daunted by the idea of teaching moves from a book—after all, it's so different from a live class. But oftentimes when I'm teaching a room full of clients of all abilities, I find myself wishing I could hand them a textbook so they could study up on how to get the very most out of barre3—and on their own terms. In a live class, I don't have time to go into detail about the philosophy of my program and how you can customize each posture. In the pages of this book, I can. I fully explain each setup, movement, and modification. You have more time to absorb the information and apply it to your workouts. I encourage you to take notes in the margins, discuss your aha moments with friends, and use social media to reach out to me and my instructors with questions and comments. I am a passionate educator, and I am excited to help you!

Q Can I really burn calories without cardio?

A The human body burns calories all day long, even during sleep. Cardiovascular exercise will allow you to burn extra calories, but cardio isn't limited to fast-paced workouts like running or using the elliptical machine. The moves you'll find in this book lift your heart rate enough to zap extra calories, but the benefits don't end there. These exercises also build muscle, which automatically revs your metabolism. The workout is a bit of a two-for-one: You build muscle and burn fat at the same time, making it efficient and effective.

Q What can I do right now?

A Keep reading! With these 10-minute workouts and easy recipes, you'll be moving—and losing—in no time

Raising the Barre

AUDRIE ABELL

AGE: 37   POUNDS LOST: 18.4   INCHES LOST: 8¾ *including 2 each from her waist and hips*

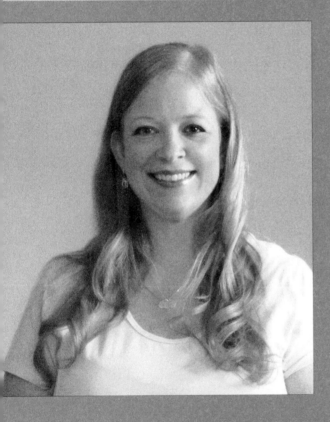

When I was younger, I wasn't huge, but I wasn't small either. In middle school, I wore a size 10 or 12, but I was also pretty active, playing softball and other sports. When I was 14, I swapped sports for dating, which wound up being a good choice for me—that year, I met the man who would eventually become my husband. Jason and I have been together for 23 years. Over that time, my weight has slowly but steadily increased, starting in college, then peaking during my two pregnancies.

A few years ago, after the birth of my daughter, Darla, I was able to lose 70 pounds through dieting, but then I got pregnant with my son, Simon, and gained 40 pounds back. I heard about Love Your Lower Body about 4 months after delivering Simon. I was feeling a little overwhelmed caring for two children, and I found that many of those healthy eating habits from before were gone. To make things easier, I usually ate whatever my daughter had left on her plate, figuring it was better than nothing. I also resorted to the always available PB&J or meat-and-cheese sandwich with chips or macaroni.

To be honest, this new plan was a little daunting at first. There were a lot of recipes that contained ingredients I didn't have at home. I had always thought I was cooking well, but this program taught me that cooking well also involves cooking a balanced meal or snack. I had spent my fair share of time in the produce department prior to this program, but now I have a greater appreciation—not to mention more space in my cart—for so many more veggies and fruits. I also do not consider myself an "exercise person." I've done a few fitness DVDs but could never get into a regular routine or even a partial routine—it's hard to put myself or my fitness first. As a mom, when my children need to be fed, bathed, cuddled, or entertained, that is my priority.

What made this program different for me was the flexibility. I can't tell you the number of times I fit in a workout while holding my son or being shadowed by my daughter—they really got into "helping" me work out. But my favorite workouts were the ones I did in complete silence, after everyone else had gone to bed. I could close my eyes during these workouts and really focus on my breathing and form.

It's amazing to me to think that just 8 weeks ago I had 18 more pounds on my frame—that's basically what my son Simon weighs, and he's starting to feel heavy! My whole family has remarked on my weight loss, and my husband has started teasing me about needing to get pants that actually fit. I do love that I am fitting into a smaller pant size and am already on my way to the next size down . . . woo-hoo!

I feel so much more energized than before and have found that eating a lot of bread or sugar really does make me more sluggish. Every time I make myself or my family a snack or a meal, I do a quick calculation to be sure it satisfies the fat-fiber-protein formula. It is becoming automatic. I'm excited and proud of these changes for myself and my family!

I LOVE MY LOWER BODY *because:*

I know I am shaping it to fit the healthier and slimmer image I have in my mind, one day at a time. I have more strength and endurance and am planning to improve even more.

Chapter 2

The SCIENCE of *Small* MOVEMENTS

"NO PAIN, NO GAIN." "BE IN IT TO WIN IT." "GO BIG OR GO HOME." THESE limit-pushing phrases can be motivating at the start of a fitness program, but when life gets hectic, I'd wager that most of us are more inclined to go home than go big. You may start a new exercise routine with a bang, putting in long hours at the gym and pushing your body beyond its limits, all in the name of getting a good workout. But after a few weeks (or, let's not kid ourselves, days), the stress on your body and mind can cause your fitness habit to fizzle well before you see lasting results. That's one reason at least half of all exercisers quit within 6 months of starting a new program, according to researchers at the University of Georgia.[1] People want a workout that's fun, that keeps their attention, and that makes their body look and feel good. Take away any of these things and a workout is going to be hard to stick to.

Traditional exercise left me feeling exhausted, not energized. Working out was no longer fun, and I wasn't getting the results I wanted, which was a trim and flexible body. That's why I decided to innovate, to be my own guinea pig, and create a workout that truly worked for me. I needed something that wouldn't trigger my chronic back pain and that would finally torch the last of my stubborn postpregnancy fat.

I began to research the best ways to tone the body. I studied different exercise disciplines that produced the kind of body I was after: both feminine and strong. I worked with doctors, physical therapists, yogis, dancers, anatomy experts, and bodyworkers. Some of the information was old news—such as the importance of muscle mass for burning fat, or the necessity of both strength training and aerobic activity for best health. But some of what I found surprised me—such as how important managing stress is for weight loss. All of the things I learned during this period of discovery influenced the development of barre3 and, consequently, Love Your Lower Body, which has proven to be safe, effective, and easy to do yet just as results-oriented as other forms of exercise.

Small Movements, Big Results

Whether you do barre3 moves in a studio or at home with the help of this book, you'll move in such a way that you slim, shape, and lift your body. Your muscles will get toned, but there's no fancy choreography, no jumping, and no large space or special gear required. In barre3 studio classes, we use a ballet barre. At home, all you need is a stable waist-height surface and a little room to move. This is a simple program that you can do anywhere.

The exercises you do during this plan will change depending on the day and week, but each and every Love Your Lower Body workout utilizes our signature three-step formula: First, you hold a position. Then you layer on small 1-inch movements. Finally, you add in larger motion. You stay in each posture for about a minute—just long enough to tax the muscles—and then move on. Let's take a closer look.

1. Holds

Every exercise starts with an isometric hold, which essentially means you find the starting position then stay there without moving. I begin with a hold because pausing before you move gives you a chance to ensure your alignment is correct. For each pose, I tell you exactly where your knees, hips, and shoulders should be. But the real power of the hold is in the way it makes your muscles fire. You don't move during a hold, yet your muscles often fatigue more quickly than they would while jumping or running.

It continues to humble me how challenging simply holding a posture is. I became inspired by this type of training when I deepened my personal yoga practice. In a typical yoga class, you might hold a pose such as Warrior II or Downward Facing Dog for several minutes at a time. By the time you get out of the pose, your muscles are fatigued, but you never even moved! I took the idea of these yoga holds and integrated them into my program. Here is why these isometric holds work.

- Holding gives you time to connect your mind to your body, focusing on proper alignment and stabilizing your core, in order to get the most out of a posture.

- Small changes in body placement can affect how well an exercise works, so it's important you get into the right position each time. Proper alignment can also keep you safe from injury by putting less pressure on the joints.

- Staying still strengthens your muscles continuously, since you are not taking breaks for muscle recovery. As you engage your muscles to stay in the posture, you tax both the large and the small stabilizer muscles. During this isometric contraction, you are able to recruit more muscle fibers all at once.

- Holding your muscles at midcontraction, their strongest point, allows you to increase your strength and endurance without having to add weight or to move. For example, a barre3 squat begins where your knees are already partway bent, which means your muscles are firing in a position where they are neither stretched nor shortened.

2. Small 1-Inch Movements

After we've gotten the attention of all of your muscles with a hold, we layer on movement that works the body in our signature 1-inch small range of motion. Behold "the Power of the Inch."

- By moving your body just 1 inch, you get even deeper into the muscles, pushing your limits and maintaining the muscular contraction until you can no longer hold it. This process is called reaching failure. When you reach failure, you are transforming the body and breaking plateaus.

- Because you are moving only 1 inch, you can keep the control and the benefits you established in your isometric hold. Why is control important when moving? When you move mindfully—instead of with momentum—you tone and shape throughout the duration of the exercise, not just on the way up or down.

- By moving just 1 inch, you can stay in the posture longer and for a higher repetition of movement. Repetition allows you to go deep in each posture to better target trouble areas. Plus, the longer you work, the more calories you burn.

- The controlled 1-inch movement creates fluidity of motion and heat in your body. Staying in an isometric hold with proper form is hard to do. The body will naturally start to lock up and tighten in an unhealthy pattern if you stay for too long. By adding on a 1-inch movement, you warm the body just enough so that you can keep a feeling of ease and the integrity of the posture without losing the strength and endurance benefits of a true hold.

- Staying in a posture for an extended period of time requires you to use your core to stabilize your posture. Even if you are doing small and controlled 1-inch leg lifts to target your glutes, you're also getting an effective abdominal workout.

3. Large Dynamic Movements

After completely taxing the muscles in our isometric hold and small 1-inch range of movement, we flush out the body with dynamic large range of motion. With this type of movement, for example, you might fully bend and completely straighten your legs instead of moving just 1 inch in the middle of a squat. Here's why this third step is so important:

- Dynamic movement increases the heart rate and increases blood-flow to the muscles. This energizes the body by infusing the muscles with fresh oxygen and nutrients, allowing you to go longer and burn more calories.

- During your isometric and small range of movement, you established good form, stability, and a mind-body connection. But you usually don't move in 1-inch increments throughout your day. Your body is meant to move big—leaning to pick up a dropped pen, squatting to tend your garden, or reaching to get a bowl from a high cabinet. This dynamic movement is translatable to how you really move in life; by layering on dynamic movement after you've found control and strength, it reinforces moving in a smart and functional way all day long.

- Working the muscles in a full range of motion creates a long, lean, and limber physique.

Dynamic movement isn't the only way to lengthen the body with large movement. This program also includes targeted stretches that release the muscle, lengthen us back out, and prepare the body for the next round of exercises. Stretching is an important part of barre3. You'll learn your first round of stretches during Week 1. I suggest specific times to stretch, but if you'd like to do even more stretching, go right ahead!

The Key Research Behind This Proven Program

This signature three-step formula helps you lose weight and shapes and tones your entire body. As simple as it sounds, my method is based on a lot of research. Here are just some of the fitness findings that have influenced barre3 and the Love Your Lower Body plan.

Major Muscles Benefit from Strong Stabilizers

Most fitness formulas focus on what I call the "outer body"—the body you see in the mirror. Traditional workouts tend to strengthen your major muscles, including your quadriceps, glutes, and biceps, because more muscle mass automatically leads to more calorie-burning. Although growing these big muscles increases metabolic rate, it's the deeper stabilizing muscles—such as the paraspinals or the serratus anterior, which both support the core—that play a big part in protecting your joints and creating a toned body. These less dominant muscles properly align the body and help you move safely all day. By using isometric holds and 1-inch movements to work the major muscle groups midcontraction, you are forced to engage the stabilizers in a way that jogging or a traditional aerobic workout never does. Once your major muscle groups reach fatigue, the stabilizers kick in to help you stay strong and steady. In this way, your moves work strategically to use both the stabilizers *and* the major muscles. This combination creates the long, lean lines of a dancer with the strength and power of an athlete.

Using Body Resistance Gets Results Quickly and Simply

Early in my career, I learned from trainers, fitness instructors, sports scientists, and my own experience that many of the most effective exercises are ones that work the full body without the need for props or gear. Things like squat jumps, planks, and burpees (which combine a squat jump and a plank) tone the full body, fast. The body's own resistance is all it takes to get a complete workout, if you're creative.

In this program, you'll find that you work all of your muscles without any fancy gadgets or machines. Instead, we take a back-to-basics approach, gathering some of the most effective moves from fitness, dance, Pilates, and yoga and working in plenty of modifications and alternatives that make the moves safe and effective for anyone. This program is full of new variations of tried and tested moves that are proven to build endurance and strength with your own body weight. In a typical Love Your Lower Body workout, you might perform a standard plank, stay low in a lunge, or drop down into a modified squat. All of these exercises work your muscles to the max without any special equipment.

Of course, I'm not totally averse to props. Most of my barre3 class workouts use a ballet barre, and you at home have the option of using my core ball for certain exercises. I love this inflatable 9-inch-diameter ball—it's easy to travel with and adds resistance to certain moves, toning your inner thighs during squats or helping you get deeper into abs work. While you are still using primarily body weight to fuel your workouts, the ball can help you extract more from some moves, which can lead to faster results. I also offer the option of using light handheld weights—usually 1- or 2-pounders—during arm exercises. But because Love Your Lower Body calls for high repetitions—we may do 30 biceps curls in a row—you can get a great workout simply by using the resistance of your arms, no weights required.

Complex Exercises Maximize Time and Effort

Complex exercises—ones that train multiple body parts and muscles at the same time—allow your body to multitask. By doubling up on training areas, you can reduce the time you spend exercising. That's why my favorite exercises target more than just one muscle at a time. This type of training will keep your full body challenged throughout the workout, and it can help improve your muscle coordination and endurance.

In this program, you'll find you're almost never working just one individual muscle. You may be focused on your legs during a certain move, but you're probably working your seat, too. While toning your seat, you're also targeting your core. When working your core, chances are you're activating all four layers of abdominals at once. By working a combination of muscle groups with each move, you'll get the most workout in the least amount of time.

Strength Routines Can Double as Cardio Workouts

Conventional exercise training says that you can either strength train or do a cardio workout. But there are ways to do both at the same time. Things like circuit training, kettlebell workouts, and even water aerobics all build muscle mass while raising the heart rate and the calorie burn. You get the benefits of both types of exercise in one workout, which ultimately saves time and simplifies your to-do list.

The Love Your Lower Body routines are based on the same principle, allowing you to strengthen and tone while boosting your calorie burn. This is how it works: By moving from pose to pose, you'll get a nonstop workout with no built-in breaks, which helps keep the heart rate elevated continuously. (Of course, I encourage you to rest when needed.) You'll move from small to large movements as you progress through each pose. The small movements boost the heart rate, and the larger ones cause it to soar, sending you into a true aerobic zone. It's similar to interval training, where you get a little breathless and then have a chance to recover.

Moderate Activity Is Best for Zapping Belly Fat and More

When it comes to dropping extra weight, study after study has shown that aerobic activity works. People who elevate their heart rate burn more calories per workout compared to those who just lift weights, and the aerobic exercisers also work off more belly fat. Eliminating this extra weight around the waist—called visceral fat—is extremely important: When fat accumulates in the belly, it increases your risk of all sorts of health problems, from type 2 diabetes to heart disease to certain types of cancer. But aerobic activity can vary greatly in intensity, from slow walking to running at an all-out sprint. Which of these is best for improving health? According to sports scientists, somewhere right in the middle.

Moderate activity, which the American College of Sports Medicine categorizes as working at between 40 and 60 percent of your maximum heart rate, presents a host of health benefits. It's the intensity that's most associated with reducing anxiety, and it's also proven to help reduce the risk of disease, increase longevity, and ease the symptoms of arthritis, according to the Centers for Disease Control and Prevention. Plus, it's an intensity that actually feels good to do. You're working hard enough to feel like you're exercising, but you're not exerting so hard that you're completely out of breath. You should be able to speak in full sentences during moderate activity and end a workout feeling energized, not exhausted.

Brisk walking and jogging count as moderate activity, and so does barre3. During a typical Love Your Lower Body workout, you'll raise your heart rate some, but not to the point that you feel as if you're running on a treadmill. You'll hold poses long enough to make sure your muscles are working, and then you'll start to move, increasing the aerobic challenge while also building lean muscle mass. Over time, training your heart in this way can improve your circulation and make you breathe more efficiently, both of which are markers of good health.

EXERCISING TO BEAT OSTEOARTHRITIS

Joint pain afflicts about 30 percent of the population at any given time, according to the Centers for Disease Control and Prevention (CDC), and knee pain accounts for more than half of those complaints. Women, in particular, are at risk for knee problems, and osteoarthritis (OA), or the wearing down of cartilage between the joints, is a major source of this discomfort. According to the CDC, one in every two people will someday be afflicted with knee OA, a painful condition that can limit mobility and cause increased inflammation.

But relief may be only a few workouts away. Hundreds of studies have shown that exercise—in particular, strength training for the muscles that support the knee joints, including the quadriceps, the hamstrings, and the associated stabilizers—can reduce the pain that comes with OA *and* make everyday tasks like walking down the stairs seem easier. One study, from the *Journal of the American Medical Association,* found that regular strength training led to a 12 percent reduction in pain and helped people with OA move better all day long, from getting in and out of the car to simply walking more quickly.[2]

Because the Love Your Lower Body workouts are designed to strengthen the muscles that support the knees, this program may help you find relief from knee pain. Several women who were part of the Love Your Lower Body test panel started the program with knee problems. Most had reduced symptoms after just a few weeks of exercise. They often worked a little bit higher—keeping their knees bent above a range of movement that felt painful—but many reported starting to work lower and without any discomfort as they gained strength. This type of work helped heal my knee problems, too: By strengthening and balancing the muscles around the joint, my once-tender knees now feel fine, even when I'm walking in heels or down hills and stairs.

Both Concentric and Eccentric Muscle Contractions Are a Must

Imagine yourself doing a biceps curl. As you bend your elbow and lift the weight toward your shoulder, your biceps (the muscles at the front of your arm between your elbow and shoulder) flex and naturally get shorter. In scientific terms, this shortening is known as a concentric muscle contraction, and it's the way most workouts build muscle. Now imagine lowering the weight. There are two ways to do this: If you simply relax your biceps, the weight will drop back to the starting position. That's what a lot of people do—they work for only half of each repetition. But what if you were to actively resist the pull of gravity as you lowered the weight? You would also be toning your biceps as your arm extends, working the muscles as they get longer, too. Engaging your muscles as they lengthen is known as an eccentric muscle contraction, and it's an important phase of movement that most people skip.

By engaging the muscles with both concentric and eccentric contractions, you get twice the toning because you are working your muscles in both directions. Another way to think about pairing these two types of muscle contractions is to envision staying engaged through an entire exercise. For example, to do a biceps curl, you would pull the weight in and then push it away—you work both ways, so there's no resting. The same applies to the leg movements. We may ask you to lower your hips 1 inch, then to lift back up, making that small shift in position active and controlled on both the up and the down.

A Powerful Core Can Safeguard Your Body

In Pilates, the core is referred to as the body's "powerhouse" because in many ways it's the place where all of your movement—from kicks to reaches—originates. A strong core will help you move better and can even bring about pain relief. If you suffer from lower-back pain like I do, one of the first things a physical therapist will prescribe is abdominal exercises. After pregnancy, retraining the abs is incredibly important—without a strong center, it's hard to bend, lift, twist, and carry. Strong abs can even improve your athletic abilities: If you're looking to better your golf swing, your tennis game, or your skill as a skier, abs training can help.

All barre3 moves take the core into consideration. During a typical leg exercise, you won't be training only your hamstrings and quadriceps,

EXERCISING TO BEAT BACK PAIN

Almost everyone I know has experienced back pain at one time or another. In fact, a recent Centers for Disease Control and Prevention survey found that 28 percent of the population had suffered from back pain in the previous 3 months alone, making it one of the most common complaints among adults.

I am part of this statistic. As a fitness professional, I used to be ashamed of my lower-back pain. In my mind, I was doing everything right: I had a regular exercise routine, including a vigorous yoga practice, and yet my back would flare up and bring me to my hands and knees. This humbling experience combating my back pain gave me empathy and a real drive to help other people discover a way to exercise that challenged and healed the body. I have studied the back and seen countless specialists ranging from spine surgeons to chiropractors to physical therapists to acupuncturists. The one thing all these professionals agree on is the importance of keeping the body in motion and finding exercises that support the spine.

There's an especially strong connection between core work and decreased back pain. Strong abs reduce pressure on the spine: When your belly bulges forward (usually due to a lack of strength and excess fat), your lower back may get pulled out of alignment, bowing forward and causing the gel-filled discs between the vertebrae to squish and bulge. If you regularly sit, walk, and stand in this position, it's only a matter of time before back pain develops. But if you work to shed fat while training your abs to draw in and support the weight of your torso, your lower back will have less pressure on it, thus staying straight and pain free.

you'll also be training your abs to engage and draw in, lengthening your lower back and firming your core in the process. Throughout class, I like to emphasize the action of hugging your waistline in—sort of like the action of cinching an imaginary corset around your waist. By drawing the abs in, you keep your core active and take extra pressure off the lower back. You may also improve your posture so that you stand with more grace and alignment than before. You might even get taller! With strong abs, the spine literally stretches out to its full length.

Using a Barre for Balance Can Help You Stand on Your Own

You'll find a waist-high ballet barre in every barre3 studio, but when you do Love Your Lower Body at home, all you need is a kitchen counter or a dining room chair. If you look around, you'll find that there are a ton of sturdy, stable things that can stand in as a barre. At the park, I hold on to the back of a bench in place of a barre. At work, I use my desk.

The ballet barre (or your counter) is there to assist in balancing the body. If you're standing in a challenging position, it can help to have some-thing stable to hold on to until you're ready to balance on your own. I also use the barre as a prop to modify postures inspired from other traditions, including yoga and functional training. You might do a plank with your hands pressing down on the barre or a squat with your hands pulling up on the barre. These variations are fun, and they also change the move-ments in two very important ways.

1. In balance postures, I use the barre to find length in the body and to gain the confidence needed to go deeper into postures. Don't think of the barre as a crutch when you balance; instead, think of it as a way to train your core and stabilizing muscles to give your body grace, length, and improved posture. Balance naturally declines with age, but if you focus on training your balance, you may stand steadier all day long.

2. I also use the barre to support postures that are usually done on the floor, such as pushups and planks. By working at the barre,

you'll put less pressure on areas of the body that are vulnerable, such as the wrists, shoulders, neck, lower back, and knees. You'll also be able to hold a position for longer and really focus on form. Because these poses are less weight bearing at the barre, we do more reps, which will help you develop long, lean muscles.

The Power of 10

I am thrilled with the results barre3 workouts have given me and my clients, but there's one really unique thing that makes the Love Your Lower Body workouts even more accessible and effective than my standard program: the way these routines are organized into 10-minute toning blocks. By arranging your workouts into small chunks—done all at once or throughout the day—you reap a ton of benefits. Here's what makes 10-minute routines not only appealing but preferable to traditional workouts:

"10" Is Convenient

How many times have you skipped a workout because you didn't have an hour to devote to exercise? If you're like most people, the answer is probably in the double or triple digits. Too little time is one of the main reasons people give for not exercising. Even a 30-minute workout takes a lot longer than half an hour. You have to change into and out of exercise clothes, and if you break a sweat, you may need to shower, too. All of these add time onto your training.

But regardless of how pressed for time you are, you almost always have an extra 10 minutes. Ten minutes is one less tap of the snooze button. It's the amount of time you need to kill while waiting for a pot of water to boil. It's the time you spend on hold on the phone while waiting for a human operator. There are tons of opportunities all day to multitask and move more. These wasted minutes could be better spent with a little extra exercise. And because you don't need to change clothing for these workouts or even root out any fitness tools, 10 minutes is truly all you need.

This shortened schedule was a hit with the Love Your Lower Body test panelists. "Ten minutes goes by fast," said Frayn Masters. "I mostly did 10 first thing in the morning, or just before bed. Oftentimes, one 10-minute workout led to another, and another." For a lot of people, the first 10 minutes of a workout are the hardest. After that, it's easy to keep going.

"10" Breaks Up Your Sitting Time

I will never forget hearing my colleague and friend Mike Clark, a physical therapist and the CEO of the National Academy of Sports Medicine, give a lecture on the dangers of sitting. He made the point that while exercise is beneficial, it's still not healthy to work out for 60 minutes and then sit for the other 23 hours of the day. All of that sedentary time—sitting in a car, at a desk, on a couch—cancels out some of the health benefits of exercise.

BODY BALANCE

strive to always create exercises that balance the body. Why is this important? Because the life we live constantly takes our bodies out of balance, which leads to all kinds of health issues ranging from weight gain to chronic pain.

Take sitting, for example. Because the majority of people sit all day long, the muscles at the front of the body are quite tight. As your shoulders slouch forward, your chest muscles start to pull in, overstretching the muscles in your back; with your legs bent at 90 degrees from your hips, your hip flexors stay in a shortened position for much of the day. Imbalances like these—where one muscle group is short and tight and the muscles on the opposite side of the body are overextended and underworked—can pull you out of alignment.

Barre3 moves are designed to bring the body back to a place of strength, balance, and alignment. Because so many people spend a lot of time sitting, the moves work to stretch and open the chest and hip flexors while strengthening the upper back and glutes. This combination of strength and stretch is the key to body balance and improved posture for long-term results.

Your metabolism slows when your body is inactive, and your blood sugar can stay elevated, putting you at greater risk for obesity and type 2 diabetes. Inactivity can increase fatigue, cause your joints to stiffen, and weaken your muscles, particularly those related to good posture. No matter how hard you work out, if a short period of exercise is all the activity you fit in that day, it can seriously hamper your health and your weight-loss efforts.

There is scientific evidence to support the benefits of breaking up your day with activity, but I learned this lesson the hard way. Early in my fitness journey, I used to be confused about why I had stubborn belly bloat and an achy lower back—after all, I was exercising for at least 60 minutes daily and eating healthily. But after hearing Dr. Clark talk, I adopted the idea of moving more all day and noticed a big shift. My back became pain free, and my digestion improved significantly. I had more energy and a clearer mind.

By spreading your workouts throughout the day, you automatically break up your sitting time. Sports scientists suggest standing up every 20 to 60 minutes; by making a couple of these standing breaks active 10-minute workouts, you'll spend less time in a chair, and you may start to move more naturally, getting out of your seat more frequently all day long. (Read about other ways to move more in Chapter 10.)

"10" Burns More Calories

Spending less time sitting can keep your fat-burning enzymes active, which automatically boosts metabolism. Simply standing burns more calories than sitting—and exercising burns even more calories—so any time spent out of your chair will be good for your waistline. But there are several other reasons mini-workouts are good for weight loss. One main factor has to do with a complex body process sports scientists call afterburn, which basically means the number of calories your body burns *after* exercise.

During a typical workout, your metabolism increases during exercise, burning more fat and calories as your heart rate elevates and your muscles work. But this elevated rate of metabolism doesn't drop off immediately after exercise. Instead, it slowly decreases over the next several hours. You may burn the same number of calories during a 30-minute workout as you would during three 10-minute workouts, but because the three periods of afterburn often last longer than the afterburn from a single session of exercise, you could easily zap more calories in the long run.

For test panelist Margueritte Kim, learning that, physiologically, 10 minutes of exercise at a clip throughout the day would bring the same—or better—results as a longer workout was a real game changer. "I no longer had or wanted an excuse not to squeeze in a workout," said Kim. "Anyone—everyone—has 10 minutes a few times a day to do something that will improve their health."

"10" Decreases Appetite

Another reason mini-workouts contribute to weight loss has to do with appetite. A study from the University of Glasgow in Scotland found that taking short walks before mealtime actually made people feel less hungry when they sat down to eat.[3] A short stint of gentle activity caused people to eat less during meals, not more. Scientists aren't sure why brief bouts of exercise before mealtime have this effect—it might be purely physiological or it may also be psychological—but it's just one more reason that these 10-minute toning blocks can put you on target for your weight-loss goals.

"10" Sounds (and Feels) Easy

Ten minutes of exercise isn't daunting, and for many people, it may not even sound like a real workout. That's what I learned from the test panelists who tried this plan. Several of them admitted to completely dreading exercise. But because these mini-workouts were so short, so simple, and so easy to do anytime, they didn't feel like typical fitness sessions. So rather than putting off the workouts, these women actually started to look for times to fit in exercise. The workouts felt accessible, even though the panelists were burning major calories and building lots of lean muscle mass. This feeling of ease may also have an effect on appetite and weight loss: If you don't feel like you're wearing yourself out with a long workout, you may not be tempted to increase your food intake, which can be a side effect of lengthy and challenging workouts.

"10" Helps You Focus

When you hit that afternoon slump, 10 minutes can come and go without much to show for it. It's easy to spend that amount of time—or, for some of us, a lot longer—surfing the Web, updating social media, or simply staring off into space. Those distractions are fun in the moment, but none of them impacts your day in a meaningful way. If you were to spend those 10 minutes exercising, you'd get all of the previously mentioned physical benefits, and you'd also get some mental benefits. Any exercise can help prevent age-related memory problems, and according to a study from the University of Illinois at Chicago, 10 minutes of exercise is enough to help bring back your focus and improve your concentration.[4] That's what researchers found when they asked 80 college students to memorize a list of words. Half of the group went on a brisk walk before the task; the other half sat down to watch a slide show. When asked what they recalled, members of the active group remembered 25 percent more than those of the inactive group.

"10" Melts Stress

Ten minutes appears to be enough time to melt away stress, according to a study in the *Journal of Physiological Anthropology and Applied Human Science*.[5] But the women in the Love Your Lower Body test panel didn't need a sports psychologist to tell them this: They naturally began to do the 10-minute routines during the most stressful parts of their days, such as when a frustrating e-mail pinged in their in-box, because the exercise helped them feel calmer and more in control. Taking an active 10-minute break gives you time to put a trying situation in perspective and acts like a form of moving meditation. By counting reps, focusing on your breath, and trying to move with precision, you may have an easier time shaking off stressors. Don't be surprised to find that you also have more energy after each 10-minute workout. A lot of the test panelists also used Love Your Lower Body routines to help beat fatigue.

"10" Creates Variety

Sports scientists agree that after following the same routine for 6 to 8 weeks, your body and mind will get bored, making the workout less effective. Because your muscles become used to the challenge, each repetition gets easier. But small variations are enough to eliminate this problem and keep your muscles and mind engaged. The design of this program—where you regularly change routines and add new moves— guarantees that your body isn't bored. Your 10-minute workouts can be shuffled in different ways, combining moves that focus on different parts of your body and that challenge your mind to keep up. You'll be able to design your own workout patterns so you'll never get bored.

"10" Is Enough to Improve Your Health

On some days of the plan, you'll exercise for three or four 10-minute blocks; on other days, you'll only do one 10-minute session. This may not sound like a lot, but regularly doing as little as 10 minutes a day can help your body perform at its peak condition. In fact, exercising for just 10 minutes right after a meal can help protect you from type 2 diabetes. According to a study from the Mayo Clinic, a short session of activity right after eating can halve the amount of sugar found in the blood, which greatly reduces your risk of developing type 2 diabetes.[6] For people who are already living with either type 1 or type 2 diabetes, short exercise sessions after meals can help minimize the need for extra insulin.

But there's more: A study from Pennington Biomedical Research Center at Louisiana State University found that 10 minutes a day was all it took to improve cardiovascular health.[7] Research from the Cleveland Clinic found that regular 10-minute workouts helped chronic pain sufferers find relief.[8] A third study, this one from the National Cancer Institute, found that just 10 minutes of daily fitness was enough to add nearly 2 years to your life.[9]

My hope is that all of this information is enough to convince you to follow the Love Your Lower Body plan from start to finish. But if you get off track, aim to fit in at least 10 minutes a day. Even that small amount of exercise is enough to make a big impact on your health.

Raising the Barre

CHRISTINA POST

AGE: 32   **POUNDS LOST:** 15.2   **INCHES LOST:** 12 *including 4 from her waist and 2 from her hips*

I was always strong and athletic. I grew up skiing and lifting weights and spending a lot of time being active. But about 13 years ago, as a sophomore in college, I broke my leg during the first varsity ski race of the year. The injury was pretty major—it took more than a year and a number of screws and rods to mend. Needless to say, I did not spend a lot of time working out during that period, which led to a weight gain of about 15 pounds. I spent the next several years working with personal trainers, counting calories, and running endlessly on the elliptical, all with little result.

Three years ago, I moved to a place where I could spend more time in the outdoors. I was really happy, but I wasn't going to the gym or watching what I ate. My boyfriend and I went on a lot of hikes, but we also ate a lot of kid-friendly foods to satisfy his 7-year-old son, which took a toll on my waistline. I was about 20 pounds heavier than I like to be. A work friend suggested I sign up for the Love Your Lower Body test panel, and I'm so glad I did.

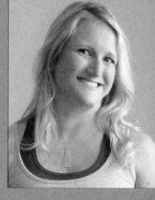

The food on the plan was my biggest surprise. The recipes were delicious, and the concept behind the eating formula was easy to grasp. I could adopt it when we ate out, which was more often than I realized. I sometimes struggled to find time for the prep work, and it was hard to explain to my boyfriend's son why I was being a "picky eater," but after a little trial and error, I found several recipes that worked really well for us all.

I absolutely loved the option to break up the workouts. Being able to do a 10- or 20-minute workout in the morning, then doing 10 at work and 10 when I got home, was easy. I found time to exercise on busy days and even in the middle of the woods while on vacation. The movements reshaped my muscles in ways that no trainer or cardio ever has. For the first time in decades, I have room in the thighs of my jeans. I was able to fit into the dress I wore to my dad's wedding back in 2000—and it was even big on me in the hips, waist, and thighs!

This program has given me the body I used to struggle so hard for. I love the energy I have and the way I can make the workouts and the food work for me. I have gotten so many compliments on how I look. And because I don't always have the best body image, having before and after pictures has really made me see how far I came in 8 short weeks!

I L♥VE MY LOWER BODY *because:*

It finally fits into pants with room to spare around my quads. I have so much more confidence now in the way I look. It feels fantastic!

Chapter 3

The LOVE Your LOWER BODY DIET

LET ME START OFF THIS CHAPTER BY TELLING YOU ONE VERY IMPORTANT thing: I love food. When I discover a tasty recipe that nourishes the body, I'm excited to share it with friends, family, and my barre3 community. Abby Fammartino, a very talented chef and the owner of Abby's Table, in Portland, Oregon, who contributed recipes to this book, shares this passion. Her mission is to make healthy meals that are an "everyday celebration." I love this idea of celebrating food whenever I eat, whether it's toasting my kids with breakfast smoothies before they rush off to school or having a fun potluck with my best friends. Even though we call the nutrition portion of Love Your Lower Body a "diet," I don't want you to feel limited or denied. I want you to enjoy food as much as you do now, and maybe even learn to love it more.

I grew up eating whole foods. Even though my family struggled financially for most of my childhood, my mom made eating whole, balanced, nutritious meals a priority. She grew some of our food and prepared meals that were dense in nutrients but easy on the pocketbook. We ate a mostly plant-based diet with whole foods like rice, veggies, and beans. When we ate meat, it was usually a special occasion like Thanksgiving. She always ordered a hormone-free and organic turkey from our local butcher—even back in the 1970s! On my birthdays, my stepdad and I would pick the ripe blackberries that grew behind our house and make a homemade cobbler instead of a birthday cake. Decades later, this tradition holds strong in my family. Even on my wedding day, we served local blackberry cobbler in place of cake. But my mom's values didn't always stick for me. There were many years that I experimented with all kinds of different foods and diets. I forced myself to drink diet soda in college because some of my girlfriends did and I thought I was missing out on something. I remember counting calories and going on a fat-free diet of pretzels and frozen yogurt. I also remember how little energy I had and how frustrating it was to be carrying around a bloated belly and an extra 15 pounds.

Fast-forward to my life today. I'm a mother of two children raising them the same way my mom raised me. After experimenting with different eating styles, I love that the diet I was raised on is the one I've come back to. This is the way of eating that makes me feel amazing in my own skin. My body is light and my energy is boundless. Best of all, I'm not alone! Eating real food—food that grows on trees and vines and in the earth—is once again becoming popular because it makes you feel and look great. An increasing number of friends, colleagues, and clients share my passion for eating this way to feel nourished in the short and long term. I hope you will, too.

Firm Up with Whole Foods

If I were to sum up the guidelines for this way of eating in a few short words, it would be this: Eat whole foods. Whole foods are those that have been processed or refined as little as possible and are free of additives and preservatives. Whole foods are natural foods that haven't been tampered with between harvest and consumption. Vegetables and fruits, whole grains, beans and nuts, and lean proteins are available in this wholly unchanged state. Whole foods don't have added sugars. They haven't had the fat extracted or other nutrients added. Whole foods are the types of things you might buy at a farmers' market—fresh leafy greens, ripe pieces of fruit, hand-ground almond butter, whole milk, lean meats, and eggs.

What makes these foods superior to processed foods—things like canned fruit, packaged cookies and chips, and TV dinners? Manufactured foods contain a lot of unnatural ingredients that our bodies simply don't recognize, including trans fatty acids, high-fructose corn syrup, and artificial colors and flavors. When you eat these things, your body doesn't know what to do with them. They eventually get lodged in your tissues, blocking necessary chemical reactions in the body. These engineered foods also contain fewer nutrients than whole foods. Because they have smaller amounts of protein and fiber, they're digested more quickly, which means you'll be hungry again sooner. Perhaps most alarming, processed foods cause spikes in your blood sugar that can send your energy levels and your mood on a roller-coaster ride.

Most processed foods are easy to spot. They come in plastic packaging, contain ingredients that are almost impossible to pronounce, and have a shelf life that's been prolonged by preservatives. Much of what you find in supermarket aisles is processed, whereas foods stocked along the perimeter of the store—fresh produce and items at the meat or seafood counter—are typically whole foods. But there are exceptions to this rule— for instance, spices are typically in the center of the store, and they offer a healthy way to add flavor to foods.

Keep in mind that some processed foods trick even the choosiest shoppers: When you reach for a food that claims to be "light," "low fat," or "fat free," the item in your cart isn't a whole food—it's been processed. Take fat-free yogurt, for example. Yogurt, on its own, is a healthy whole food. Whether Greek or regular, plain unsweetened yogurt contains a nice blend of protein and healthy fats, and it's also full of nutrients and healthy bacteria. But when the fat is removed, some of the proteins are also taken out. What you're left with is the sugar content of dairy, minus many of the essential nutrients.

In my twenties, I thought that eating fat-free foods would make me skinny and healthy. I ate all kinds of processed foods—from fat-free cookies to fat-free ice cream to fat-free cheese. These products didn't nourish me. Because the fat-free versions lacked a balance of healthy fat, fiber, and protein, they weren't satisfying or filling. In an attempt to get full, I would eat more and more of these foods, packing in empty calories that converted to unwanted pounds. Sound familiar?

One last tip for avoiding processed foods: Marketing can be misleading. Foods labeled "gluten free," "vegan," "organic," "sugar free," "natural," or "whole grains" can be just as processed and bad for you as more obvious junk food choices. Read all the ingredients on the back of the package before you put it in your cart. You might find that the organic cereal you picked up is actually made from organic refined white flour and loaded with sugar— the same ingredients found in the cookies and cakes you are avoiding.

Foods to Phase Out

As you usher in new foods like quinoa and endive, it's time to get rid of the foods (and beverages) that have sabotaged your past weight-loss attempts, made your moods and energy levels erratic, and brought inflammation and stress into your body. Here are the not-so-fab four: the foods, drinks, and ingredients that cause so many bodies so much trouble. Simply eliminating these will do wonders; when you replace them with healthier choices, you'll only improve your results.

Alcohol: Simply put, alcohol is sugar. Drinking alcohol can greatly increase your daily calorie consumption, and it also causes a huge blood sugar spike; much of that extra energy will eventually be converted to fat. As if that wasn't bad enough, alcohol also causes inflammation, raises triglycerides, and increases your risk of diabetes (not to mention hangovers). Then there's the lowered inhibition. Have you ever noticed how hard it is to avoid snacking on processed foods after a glass of wine or a pint of beer? That's what happens when your willpower is weakened and your blood sugar crashes. Still, I know there are times when water just won't do. When I want wine, I drink sparkling water with a splash of cherry juice out of a wine glass. When beer is on my mind, I pop open a bottle of kombucha, a fermented tea that has a natural fizz.

Coffee: A lot of people I know drink their coffee "light and sweet," meaning they add a ton of sugar and cream. This turns a cup o' joe into a calorie-laden treat. But even unadulterated coffee is bad for your body. Caffeine stimulates the release of cortisol, our stress hormone, and cortisol speeds the absorption of sugar into the bloodstream. As with all blood sugar surges, the unspent energy will be converted to stored fat.

If you need an extra energy perk, I'm a big believer in green tea. It contains some caffeine—though only about a quarter of what you'll find in coffee. Plus, it has been shown to boost metabolism. Up until recently, if you had asked if I would ever give up coffee, my answer would have been simple: *No way!* I loved the ritual and the smell of a fresh brew. For more than 20 years, I had coffee every single morning. It was the first thing I thought of when I woke up. Then, about 2 years ago, when I was feeling low on energy and burnt out from head to toe, one of my instructors, Alison, gave me a Japanese full-leaf green tea. She said to steep it for only 20 seconds so it didn't get bitter. Alison is in her fifties, but I swear she looks 30, tops. Her skin glows, and she has endless energy. I decided to give her green tea a try.

At first I had the tea only every once in a while. But I soon noticed how hydrated I felt when I drank it. I bought a pretty tea mug and strainer and started to sip green tea more and more. It didn't take me long to realize that thanks to the tea, I had fewer wrinkles, glowing skin, better digestion, and sustained energy all day long. Now I almost exclusively drink green tea in place of coffee.

I don't recommend that you stop drinking coffee cold turkey—caffeine is a drug, after all, and withdrawals from it can cause unwanted side effects like headaches. Instead, I suggest decreasing your intake slowly until you get down to one cup a day. Once you get there, see if you can add in tea and eventually replace java altogether.

Gluten: You've probably heard of gluten sensitivity and gluten allergy; they're among the most talked-about health concerns right now because gluten is difficult for many people to digest, causing inflammation, blocking nutrient absorption, and disrupting the immune system. Gluten is a protein found in grains including wheat, barley, rye, and triticale and in foods such as bulgur wheat, durum flour, graham flour, kamut, semolina, and spelt. Oats are often contaminated with gluten, so avoid these, too, unless they're labeled "gluten free." Doctors believe that part of the reason this intolerance to gluten developed is because of our overconsumption of it: Gluten is commonly found in beer, breads, cakes, candies, cereals, cookies, french fries, pastas, pies, salad dressings, sauces, seasoned snacks, and soups. To reduce and eventually eliminate your gluten intake, add gluten-free grains, such as amaranth, arrowroot, buckwheat, corn, millet, gluten-free oats, quinoa, rice, sorghum, tapioca, and teff.

Refined sugar: Refined sugars include high-fructose corn syrup, sucrose, and white sugar. Most processed foods—from ice cream to pasta sauce—contain these ingredients, which cause blood sugar spikes and contribute to weight gain. High-fructose corn syrup is especially unhealthy: Some studies suggest that it is strongly linked to type 2 diabetes and that it actually causes the body to hang on to more fat than other types of sweeteners.[1] Artificial sweeteners are not a healthy alternative to refined sugars. They contain chemicals that our body does not process well.

Giving up refined sugar doesn't mean giving up sweets. Small portions of dates, figs, dried fruit, brown rice syrup, blackstrap molasses, raw honey, and pure maple syrup are okay. Stevia, which is available at most natural food stores, is another alternative to artificial sweeteners. When I want something sweet, I add dates to smoothies, molasses to oatmeal, and maple syrup to my yogurt. Occasionally giving in to your sweet tooth is okay—just remember to keep it to a minimum and always include protein and healthy fat.

Your Portion Prescription

To keep your body running at its optimal form—and to keep your metabolism going strong all day long—you need a diet that contains fat, protein,

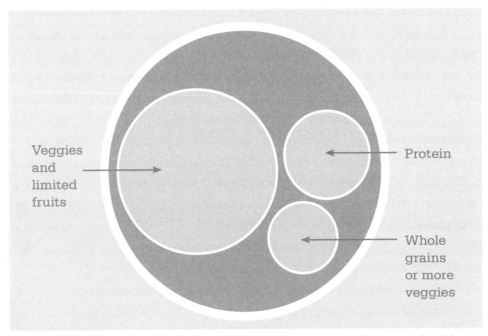

Here's what your plate should look like if you're using our formula for the right amount of protein, fat, and fiber. You'll have mostly veggies, with an emphasis on greens and limited fruit, a serving of healthy protein, and some whole grains (or more veggies). Include a moderate amount of healthy fat with each meal as well.

and fiber. These foods work in tandem to help your body digest the greatest amount of nutrients and to stabilize your blood sugar levels. In Chapter 7, you'll find recipes that will help you easily get the right balance of nutrients on your plate. Here's an explanation of how these foods contribute to a healthy diet.

Fat: You've probably heard that protein and fiber are part of a healthy balanced diet, but fat? Really? I was surprised, too. Most of us have spent years trying to avoid fat. But as I've learned from conversations with nutritionists as well as my own nutrition transformation, fat is a vital part of a healthy diet. Fat is essential for our body to absorb fat-soluble vitamins, including vitamins A, D, E, and K. Imagine you fill your plate with spinach and sweet potatoes one evening. Both vegetables contain high levels of vitamins A and K. However, you won't get the benefits of these vitamins unless you eat fat, too. Fat has been proven to help the body in numerous other ways: It improves memory, keeps hair and skin healthy, and can relieve joint pain, to name a few.

Some fats are better than others. Omega-3 fatty acids are the best. A type of unsaturated fat, omega-3s have made headlines in recent years for their anti-inflammatory properties, their role in reducing the risk of memory loss and dementia, and their power to combat heart problems. This type of fat can be found in foods like avocados, fish, olive oil, and flaxseed, and the Love Your Lower Body diet is focused on making sure you get enough of it. To get your fill of omega-3s, you might grill a piece of salmon for your entrée, top a salad with avocado slices, or sprinkle flaxseed in your smoothie. Omega-6s are another healthy fat to seek out. They're found in nuts, seeds, and whole grains. We emphasize these healthy fats over saturated fats in Love Your Lower Body.

Saturated fats are found in animal-based foods like steak, cheese, and ice cream as well as in some plant-based foods such as coconut oil. The federal government suggests limiting saturated fat to 10 percent of your daily calories. Coconut oil and whole milk yogurt are saturated fats that are a part of the Love Your Lower Body program. In moderation, these whole foods help to satiate the body and trigger hormones that tell us we're full. When I have dairy, which is a source of essential fatty acids, I make sure it's organic and hormone free. I limit my cheese consumption because it is often heavily processed and loaded with sodium. I think of cheese as something designed to add flavor but not to fill in as a main course. But when it comes to milk and yogurt, whole milk varieties are the way to go. I'd rather have you eat a little extra fat and get those nutrients than skip the fat and take in empty calories.

It is important to differentiate healthy fats from fats you should avoid altogether. Manufactured fats, such as trans fatty acids, are fats that our bodies don't recognize or know how to digest. They stay in our bodies, clogging arteries and raising bad cholesterol levels. Margarine, most fried foods, canola oil, and many packaged foods contain trans fats. If you're unsure, look for the term "partially hydrogenated" on the label—that's a dead giveaway there are trans fats in a food. This fat offers a lot of cons and no pros—that's why we'll avoid it completely.

Protein: Proteins are made up of amino acids, which are the building blocks for all of the tissues in the body, from your quadriceps muscles to the cells that line your gut. This important nutrient can be found in both animal and plant-based sources: A cup of milk has the same amount of protein as ¼ cup almonds, ½ cup cooked legumes, or a slice of lean meat. Many popular diets emphasize eating protein because of its key function of building muscle and because lean proteins actually take a lot of energy to digest: Your body burns a significant number of calories as it breaks down and absorbs protein. Proteins also help in the production of serotonin and GABA, neurotransmitters that can help stabilize your mood, which indicates why protein is important for staying happy.

Many of the recipes in this plan include animal protein, ranging from fish to lamb to eggs and dairy. These are all good sources of protein, but you can also get plenty by eating a plant-based diet. My favorite protein-rich foods are beans, nuts, seeds, and even some whole grains. If you are a meat eater, I encourage you to try vegetarian and vegan recipes from time to time to get more of these plant proteins into your diet. If you are vegan or vegetarian, try replacing the meat and dairy ingredients in the recipes with alternatives like tempeh, legumes, and nut milks such as almond or hazelnut milk. This process of trying new ways of eating will deepen what I call your *body wisdom,* your ability to listen to your body's cues as it tells you what it needs, not just what it wants. You will learn which foods truly feed you and which ones you eat out of habit. Take the time to figure out how to best feed your energy levels, your weight goals, and your values. Most importantly, keep learning how to feed your love of eating!

Fiber: One of the reasons fiber is an important component of this diet—and many others—is because it's filling. Fiber takes up a lot of space in the stomach, and because it's slow to digest, you'll feel full longer. We need fiber for digestion to keep the food moving through—and eventually out of—our bodies. Fiber also feeds the gut's healthy bacteria, which prevent unhealthy bacteria and stomach bloat.

Fiber is naturally found in complex carbohydrates such as fruits, vegetables, whole grains, legumes, and nuts. These foods keep your blood sugar stable and are full of nutrients, vitamins, and antioxidants, all of which will help your body run better. Veggies—particularly leafy greens—are my go-to source for fiber. That's why they take up a full half of the Portion Prescription plate—they fuel the body and continue to satisfy hours after eating. *Caution:* Beware of packaged high-fiber foods that are made of processed ingredients and contain lots of sweeteners. Whole foods are your best sources of fiber.

Balancing Your Blood Sugar

You've probably heard of blood sugar spikes—when sugar is rapidly absorbed into the bloodstream after a meal, causing surges of energy that come on quickly and then drop off just as suddenly, sending your energy levels, mood, and metabolism crashing. This is one thing we're trying to avoid on this plan. When you eat foods that keep your blood sugar stable, your mood and your energy levels will also remain steady and your metabolism will keep burning calories all day long.

Foods that are quickly released into the bloodstream score high on the glycemic index (GI), a scale that details the rate at which carbohydrates are converted to fuel in the body. Most processed foods score high on this index—crackers, candy, soda, and bread, for instance—and so do a handful of starchy whole foods such as bananas and baked potatoes. Getting a quick jolt of extra energy may sound like a good thing, especially when you're feeling tired. But a sudden surge in blood sugar will overload your body with energy, and when this fuel isn't used up, it is converted into fat. The inevitable blood sugar crash can result in fatigue, headaches, cravings for sugar and caffeine, and even nausea or dizziness.

The Love Your Lower Body nutrition formula is designed to balance your blood sugar levels so you lose weight and feel great. By avoiding processed foods, gluten, coffee, alcohol, and refined sugars, you automatically eliminate some of the biggest sources of blood sugar spikes. But I prefer to focus on what you get to put *in* your grocery cart versus what you need to take out. Many of my favorite whole foods score low on the GI, which means they release slowly into the body and leave you balanced and refreshed, not sugar crazed. Vegetables such as spinach, celery, and cucumbers fall into this category, as do black beans, lentils, peanuts, chickpeas, and grapefruit. These foods keep your energy levels steady all day.

Combining foods is another way to manage your blood sugar levels. Every meal, every snack, and every bite you take while following the Love Your Lower Body nutrition plan will include fiber, healthy fats, and protein. They work together to stabilize blood sugar and keep you feeling satisfied

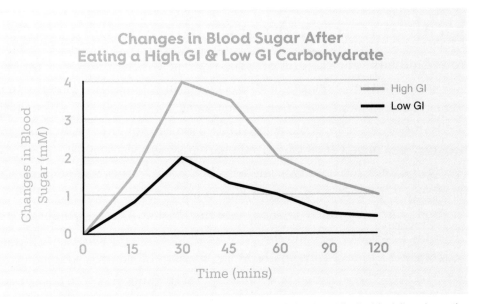

The blue line shows the spike and crash cycle of eating high-GI foods, while the black line shows the small rises and falls indicative of a healthier diet in which protein, fiber, and fat are in balance.

longer after meals. So when you eat a whole food that rates higher on the GI, such as sweet potatoes, its effects will be tempered by slower-to-digest foods like chicken, spinach, and olive oil.

The benefits of this diet go beyond weight loss; they extend to your mood, your energy levels, and even your relationships. When I began eating this way, I noticed a shift in how I felt after meals and all day long. I experienced fewer cravings, felt full longer, and found that a sense of calm and ease became my norm. Take note of all of these things as you embark on this journey. The more positive benefits you notice in all areas of your life, the easier it'll be to make this shift permanent.

Putting It All Together

On the following pages, you will find a grocery list, suggested snacks for when you're on the go, and a sample meal plan to get you started. On this plan, you'll eat three square meals each day plus one or two snacks. The recipes you choose will change from day to day, but many call for similar ingredients. The goal of this section is to show you what those ingredients are and how you can put them together for a week of delicious meals.

Grocery List

These are my favorite foods—and the ones you'll be eating the most. When in doubt, stick to this list and be sure to include foods from each category—proteins, healthy fats, and fiber—in each meal.

Proteins

(Organic and raised without growth hormones, when possible)

- Beans
- Beef
- Chicken
- Eggs
- Lamb
- Nuts
- Pork
- Seeds
- Turkey
- Whole milk, plain yogurt, and cottage cheese (on occasion)
- Wild fish*

*Wild fish have more nutrients than farm-raised fish, but if wild fish are unavailable, farm-raised fillets are the next best thing.

Healthy Fats

(Sources of omega-3 and omega-6 fatty acids, as well as mono- and polyunsaturated fatty acids)

- Nuts and nut butters (almonds, cashews, peanuts, and walnuts)
- Oils (coconut, flaxseed, olive, and sesame oils)
- Seeds (chia, ground flaxseed, hemp, pumpkin, sesame, and sunflower)

Fiber

Veggies (fresh—not canned—and organic, when possible)

- Avocados
- Beets
- Cabbages
- Carrots
- Celery
- Cucumbers
- Green beans
- Leafy greens (arugula, bok choy, chard, collards, kale, lettuces, and spinach)
- Peas
- Radishes
- Squash
- Sweet potatoes
- Tomatoes
- Zucchini

Fruits (fresh—not dried—and organic, when possible; frozen is okay)

- Apples
- Apricots
- Blueberries
- Cherries
- Dates
- Figs
- Grapefruit
- Grapes
- Oranges
- Peaches
- Pears
- Plums
- Strawberries

Whole grains

- Amaranth
- Brown or wild rice
- Buckwheat
- Gluten-free pasta (on occasion)
- Millet
- Quinoa
- Steel-cut oats

10 Grab-and-Go Snack Ideas

I've provided plenty of recipes in Chapter 7 so you can prepare delicious, healthy meals, but it's also important to have healthy snacks at the ready for when there's no time to cook. Here are my favorite grab-and-go snacks.

1. A handful (approximately ¼ cup) of almonds, walnuts, cashews, Brazil nuts, hazelnuts, pumpkin seeds, or sunflower seeds. Try a combo, as long as the ingredients add up to no more than ¼ cup.

2. A sliced apple, pear, or banana with 2 to 4 tablespoons peanut, almond, or sunflower butter

3. 1 cup sliced fresh carrots, celery, sugar snap peas, peppers, broccoli, or cauliflower dipped in ¼ cup hummus

4. 1 leaf of lettuce wrapped around an avocado slice, veggies of your choice, and an optional slice of honey-roasted turkey

5. A serving of whole grain gluten-free crackers, such as Mary's Gone Crackers, with a few slices of avocado

6. A handful of celery or carrot sticks spread with unsweetened nut or seed butter

7. ½ cup dried chickpeas with sea salt (you can roast them ahead of time and store in an airtight container)

8. ½ cup whole milk yogurt, with a handful of berries

9. Trail mix: Make your own with 3 cups raw nuts and seeds, 1 cup dried fruit or coconut flakes, and ¼ cup dark chocolate (1 serving = ¼ cup)

10. Protein Power "Barre" (see the recipe on page 282; make these ahead of time and store in the refrigerator for up to 1 week or in the freezer for up to 1 month. 1 serving = one 2 x 2-inch square.)

SAMPLE MEAL PLAN

Part of making this plan your own is choosing which meals are right for you and using the grocery list to make your own creations. But if you're looking for inspiration, here's how I organized 1 week of Love Your Lower Body recipes.

	BREAKFAST	LUNCH	SNACK(S)	DINNER
Monday	DIY Muesli (page 232)	Turkey-Avocado Lettuce Wrap (page 256)	Handful of almonds Chocolate-Hazelnut Bites (page 283)	Spicy Harvest Soup (page 238)
Tuesday	DIY Smoothie (page 226)	Spicy Harvest Soup leftovers	DIY Smoothie leftovers	Seared Tuna with Minted Quinoa Salad (page 261)
Wednesday	Savory Rice Porridge (page 234; Use leftover quinoa from Tuesday dinner.)	Tuna Niçoise Salad with Dijon Vinaigrette (page 245; Use leftover tuna from Tuesday dinner.)	Crunchy Kale Chips (page 278) ½ cup yogurt with raspberries	Lemon-Garlic Chicken and Polenta with Roasted Vegetables (page 268)
Thursday	DIY Smoothie	Polenta Salad (page 242; Use leftover polenta from Wednesday dinner.)	DIY Smoothie leftovers	Black Bean Chili (page 257)
Friday	Skinny Omelet with Greens (page 231)	Black Bean Bowl with Cumin-Lime Dressing (page 244)	Hummus and carrots	Dinner out (I stuck with grilled meat and veggies.)
Saturday	Pumpkin Spice Smoothie (page 228)	DIY Salad and Dressing (page 240)	Smoothie leftovers ½ apple with 2 Tbsp peanut butter	Foil-Wrapped Fish with Olive Vegetable Medley (page 262)
Sunday	Buckwheat Buttermilk Pancakes with Blueberries (page 236)	Grilled Fish Salad (page 246; Use leftover fish from Saturday dinner.)	Protein Power "Barre" (page 282)	BBQ with friends: Grilled salmon (protein) Grilled asparagus (fiber) Sliced avocados (fat)

The Fine Print

I'm not going to tell you the number of calories you should consume each day, because everyone's needs are different. The goal is to learn to sense your own point of satiety, where you're no longer hungry but you also aren't totally full.

Here are a few hints for getting into a healthy eating routine.

Plan ahead. Confession: I don't eat this way 365 days of the year. I splurge on my anniversary or when visiting my in-laws, and I'm happy about these "cheats." I'm not so happy about the times I go off plan simply because I forgot to pack my lunch or didn't have time to prepare a healthy dinner after a long day on the road. This is not the fun kind of bending the rules—it's the kind that brings on pangs of guilt. Do what you can to minimize your chances of being caught without a healthy option. I carry sprouted almonds in my purse, stow hummus in the fridge at work, and wash and chop all of my veggies right when I get home from the store to simplify meal prep. Take away any barriers between you and healthy foods and you'll have a much better chance of going off plan only when you want to.

Time your meals. Everybody is different, but in general most people should eat something every 3 to 5 hours. Be sure you don't get to the place where you're starving, nauseated, or having fuzzy thoughts. Long periods without sustenance are hard on the body. I recommend eating three meals plus one or two snacks each day to help keep your body at its peak. You needn't plan meals and snacks around your short 10-minute workouts. However, when you do 20 or 30 minutes of continuous exercise, I would recommend eating a small snack of protein, fat, and fiber before exercise. This will help you stay strong and energized all workout long.

Keep snacks small. I have a few words of caution about snacking: I learned the hard way that snacking can get out of control. When I first began to shift to this style of eating, I went nuts eating nuts. I munched on nuts and spoonfuls of peanut butter with gusto, and my waistline didn't budge. I was simply eating too much, more than my body needed to stay healthy and satisfied. Now I grab a small handful and limit myself to that portion along with a big glass of water. Snacks should be small, controlled portions, not real meals.

Eat early. Let's hear it for eating a healthy and hearty breakfast and lunch each day: Consuming a majority of your calories before midafternoon can actually help speed up weight loss. In a study that was published in the *International Journal of Obesity,* researchers tested how the timing of meals affected weight loss. In the 20-week study, people were assigned to eat lunch at one of two times: before or after 3:00 p.m. Those who ate earlier in the day lost significantly more weight than those who pushed back eating until later, even though both groups consumed the same number of calories.[2]

I try not to eat after 8:00 p.m., but curbing afternoon and evening eating is one thing I personally struggle with. After dinner, I often find myself wandering into the kitchen and right into my pantry. What I have learned is that I am usually just tired and need to unplug and rest. Going to food when you are tired is a natural instinct because food is associated with energy. This is why my sweet tooth takes over at night—sugar is quick energy. Now when I find myself reaching for the cookies, I instead boil a pot of water and make a giant cup of chamomile tea. This helps me unwind and ultimately have a sound night's sleep. If tea doesn't cut it, you can always add a handful of nuts, which have the mix of fiber, fat, and protein that you should aim for at every meal. Or you can try a more extreme solution one of my friends confessed to: She actually sets her home security system to sound an alarm if she enters the kitchen after a certain hour. Oh, the things we do!

Change how you eat. Sometimes it's the small stuff—like how you arrange your cabinets or the dishes you eat off of—that helps with weight loss. The food psychology gurus at the Cornell University Food and Brand Lab have pinpointed dozens of things you can do to positively change your food interactions. Here are a few of my favorite ways to get even better results from the plan.

- *During meals, keep serving dishes out of sight.* You'll be less tempted to take a second helping if it's not within reach.

- *Don't shop hungry.* When your stomach is rumbling, you're more inclined to stock your cart with high-calorie foods.

- *Place healthy foods front and center.* By setting a bowl of fruit (or nuts or veggies) on the counter or at the front of the fridge, you're more likely to snack on healthy foods.

- *Eat off of salad plates.* Like a belly-fattening optical illusion, the larger your plate, the more inclined you are to fill it.

Eat mindfully. If you eat on the go—scarfing down breakfast during the drive to work or eating your workday lunch while hunched over your computer—your body will have a harder time digesting food and extracting all the important nutrients. Your mind and body will be stuck in fight-or-flight mode, which puts your nervous system in overdrive and appears to contribute to a variety of digestive issues, including irritable bowel syndrome.

If this is you, it's time to change how you view the time you spend eating. Meals are a time to take a break from the rest of your day, not a time to multitask. This may be a new idea for you, but my goal for mealtime is to relax my body and brain and enter a parasympathetic state—basically the opposite of fight-or-flight mode. This is commonly known as the rest-and-digest state, and it leads to improved digestion and fewer tummy troubles because it provides a natural break from stress.

To get yourself into eating mode, take a break from work and all of life's busyness. Step away from your computer, TV, and phone so you can turn your focus to the food in front of you. Start your meal with a few deep breaths into your abdomen, which will help you enter that relaxed state. Once you are relaxed, take your time and chew your food well. I learned the importance of chewing from one of my advisors, the very talented functional nutritionist Andrea Nakayama. She explained that chewing is where digestion starts and is a key step to processing food for fuel versus storing it as fat. Sitting and chewing your food well allow the digestive enzymes in your mouth to work right away. Between bites, put down your utensils and savor the experience. People who eat slowly are less likely to be overweight than those who rush through a meal, according to a study in the *British Medical Journal.*[3] It can take 15 or 20 minutes for your body to signal your brain that it's been fed. If you eat a meal too quickly, your stomach gets loaded up long before your brain receives the message, often leading to overfullness.

Crowd Out Unhealthy Options

You may have noticed that I don't put a lot of emphasis on the things you shouldn't be eating on this plan. Instead, I focus on what to add to your daily diet. When you fill your belly with healthy and satisfying foods, you simply won't have room for unhealthy options and, over time, you'll naturally want them less. That's why so much of your success on this diet is about planning ahead—making your meal plan for the week, shopping for just the groceries you need, and preparing large enough batches and using leftovers to cut down on your time in the kitchen. I've given you a nutrition game plan, but it's still important to have strategies in place for skipping the foods you shouldn't eat, especially processed foods. Here are some suggestions for staying on track.

Reframe Your Thoughts

Many of us beat ourselves up for even thinking about foods on the "forbidden" list. This isn't good for your spirit, and it's also bad for your body: When you already feel guilty, you're more likely to cheat. I was speaking to Frayn Masters, one of the Love Your Lower Body test panelists, about this, and she had some amazing insight on how to react when these thoughts hit.

"When you are faced with something you really want to eat or drink, instead of thinking of it as cheating, or 'being bad,' remember that it's a normal impulse," Masters said. "So don't feel bad for having the thought or for considering giving in. Simply ask yourself, 'Do I really want to be healthier and get in better shape?' Really ask it. If the answer is yes, then you aren't saying no to that candy bar. You are saying yes to your goal, to what you really want."

I do something similar. When I want to "cheat," I repeat a mantra of sorts to remind myself that I'm in this for the long haul, that a short-term distraction isn't going to derail my diet. Some of my favorite phrases include: "Health is really important to me" and "Managing my weight is really important to me." Switching my thoughts to these phrases easily blocks out the impulse to dig into a pint of Ben and Jerry's.

Think about what *you* want from this program and how those goals support your priorities. Maybe it's a long-term goal like having more energy around your kids so you can be more present. Maybe it's a short-term goal like confidently rocking a pair of skinny jeans for your reunion. When thoughts of an unhealthy food start to pester you, drop the negative thoughts—the "I shouldn'ts"—and focus instead on what is important to you and the big picture. This will make it infinitely easier to resist those temptations.

Kick Cravings to the Curb

Cravings strike, but before you give in, I'd like you to do one thing first: Reach for a really good alternative and see if it satisfies you. When I am craving salty and crunchy, I make a big batch of kale chips. I don't limit how many I eat—they're so much better for me than the salty potato chips I used to turn to. When my kids recently made a thick strawberry milkshake with extra ice cream, I made my own version with whole milk yogurt, sweet dates, and strawberries. (You can find the recipe on page 285.) Guess what? My kids tasted it and liked it better than theirs. The point is, you can eat whole, healthy foods that satisfy your cravings.

Stick with It

When our 8-week test panel first kicked off, I could tell that the women in the group didn't believe that their cravings would go away or that their tastes and preferences would change. I saw a lot of skeptical looks when I

YOUR OUTLOOK ON EATING

Why do so many people fall into the trap of emotional eating? Why is there such a strong connection between what we eat and how we hope it will make us feel? The answers are complicated, but here are two very big reasons: First, from a very young age, most of us were taught to think of food as an appropriate reward; and second, some unhealthy foods are actually interpreted by the brain as extremely pleasurable.

Think back to your childhood. Each time you were bribed with ice cream to clean your room, you were being conditioned to think of food as something other than fuel and sustenance for your body. For parents, food is something with leverage, a bargaining chip that is just as easy to hand out as television time or similar perks.*

But the real reason this "coercion by junk food" strategy works is because sweet, high-calorie, unhealthy foods light up the reward center of the brain more than other foods, according to scientists from Duke University Medical Center.[4] The foods we crave release neurotransmitters in our brain that make us feel good. We want that sensation, so we eat the food. Cupcakes, cookies, cheeseburgers, and the like literally bathe your brain in feel-good chemicals, and the more you eat, the more you want.

There is a way to break the sugar cycle: Stop eating those foods. It sounds simplistic, but hear me out. Researchers have found that cravings for this "buzz" diminish and eventually disappear if the brain isn't regularly stimulated.[5] It's the reason most parents try to keep candy away from young children for as long as possible—you can't miss what you don't know (or remember).

*Full disclosure: As a mom, I fall right into this pattern of parenting. One time, I stuck a lollipop in my daughter's mouth to keep her quiet during a conference call—parenting can be so humbling! I think back on this moment of desperation when I'm tempted to bribe my kids—or reward myself—with food. There are so many better ways!

mentioned that I rarely thought about sugary treats and that I now actually preferred green tea to coffee. But these disbelievers experienced the same transformation I underwent when I first started this style of eating.

During the first week of the plan, the test panelists wanted plenty of reminders about why they were making different changes. They needed to know exactly why they were making this sacrifice: what was in it for them if they started to replace the unhealthy foods and drinks they were attached to with better options. But soon—within days for most of the women—they started to tell me that their cravings were disappearing. Suddenly, 8 weeks didn't seem so daunting.

It was around Week 6 that something sort of magical happened. Our conversations started to shift. Not only were the cravings gone, these women noticed that their actual preferences had started to change. They no longer thought about sugary lattes and cupcakes, and when they allowed themselves a bite or a sip of those treats, they were surprised by how overly sweet, how unnatural, how disappointing these one-time favorites tasted. Some test panelists told me that they'd started to modify the smoothie recipes to cut down on the sweetness. Others were surprised to find sparkling water more satisfying than soda. Still others admitted to loving kale. If 1 month was enough time to make the plan feel doable, 2 months was enough to make it not only second nature but also first choice.

At the start of the plan, it never once occurred to these women that the diet would stick. Many had committed to weight-loss plans before, but they admitted to counting down the moments until they could get back to their "normal" way of eating. When I started to hear about all of these changes, not just in habit but also in actual preference, I knew that what we were doing really worked. Much of what we eat is consumed simply out of habit. Detoxing from processed foods allows you to see which choices actually feel good in your body, and knowing what feels good makes establishing new habits easy. Your body will start to crave healthy choices and shun the rest. Before long, it won't even feel like a choice. It'll become automatic.

Raising the Barre

FRAYN MASTERS

AGE: 40   POUNDS LOST: 11.6   INCHES LOST: 6¾ *including 3¼ from her waist and 2¼ from her hips*

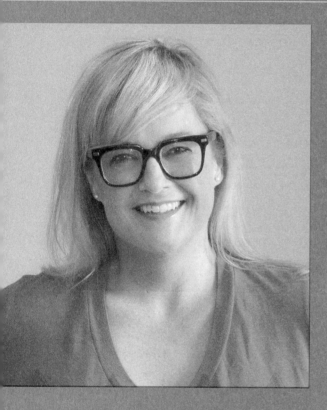

I make my living as a copywriter, producer, and performer—which I love—but one of the drawbacks of being a freelance writer is that I spend a lot of time sitting at the computer. And my hobbies involve sitting, too. Sitting to read. Sitting to watch documentaries and movies. This sedentary lifestyle combined with a few recent medical problems caused me to gain about 37 pounds over the last 4 years. I've never been small, but over this period, I became bigger than I'd ever been before. I felt uncomfortable with my appearance and disappointed that my body was not functioning as well as I know it can. I'd never felt so schlumpy or been so out of shape in my life.

I'd had enough with feeling this way, so I recently sought out a naturopath who helped balance out my digestive system. Over 5 months, I was able to shed nearly 30 pounds by eating from a plan similar to the Love Your Lower Body Portion Prescription. Because I felt so much better, I also exercised more. But then the scale got stuck. Instead of freaking out about hitting a set point, I decided to be okay maintaining for a while—my body needed a little time to adjust. Then as spring came around, I heard about the Love Your Lower Body test panel. The timing really could not have been better.

It's been amazing to learn how much I absolutely love this kind of exercise. I see myself as strong, tall, and lean like a ballet dancer when I practice on my own. When I do the small movements and the short routines, time goes by quickly, and my body feels stronger almost immediately. I'm also more energized, have the sensation of being lighter, and most definitely have better brain-power and concentration all through the day. It's life changing to feel like my body is pulling me forward rather than dragging me down.

I like that the recipes are easy to make and that this program didn't require nearly as much shopping for each meal as some of the other ones I've tried. The Love Your Lower Body plan gives instructions on how to add excitement to leftovers, which only makes it feel more doable. I have definitely found a few new favorite recipes. When I serve them to friends and family, they eat it up and comment on how delicious it is. That is big.

I lost almost 4 inches around my waist and got more toned in my arms, back, shoulders, and legs. How can I not be overjoyed about that? I feel great and confident in my clothes, and I look so much stronger and taller. But my biggest "win" was a shift to being concerned with getting my exercise in and eating well rather than being supremely focused on my weight and size. There was no unhealthy focus on the scale, just a real concentration on creating healthy habits, which is a far more peaceful way to go through life. This program helped me understand that you can love your lower body even when it's not perfect, that you can love how much stronger it is getting.

I LOVE MY LOWER BODY *because*:

It is strong. It makes me feel light, and I can spring up stairs like a youthful gazelle. When the basement door won't shut, I can kick it closed—from the core, thus not injuring myself . . . thus feeling like a badass. I am fortunate to have powerful legs that can take me great distances without even thinking about it. The more balance, flexibility, grace, and strength I gain, the more excited I get about all aspects of my life.

Chapter 4

The LOVE Your LOWER BODY Plan

HAVING READ THIS FAR, YOU ALREADY KNOW *WHY* THE LOVE YOUR LOWER Body plan works. You'll be doing the best lengthening and strengthening moves and eating nutritious and delicious recipes that boost energy and fuel your body for weight loss and strength gains. Now it's time to learn how to put it all together.

An Overview

I've hinted at some of the specifics. You're going to follow a schedule of 10-minute workouts, doing just one 10-minute session on some days and up to 40 minutes of activity on other days. You know that the moves combine muscle-building isometric holds with metabolism-boosting small and large movements. You also know that you're going to shift to eating a diet of whole foods full of protein, fiber, and healthy fats, effectively crowding out unhealthy options.

In Chapter 5, you will learn all about the 10 Transformative Minutes, the basis of the Love Your Lower Body plan. That one 10-minute workout is super-effective, but you don't have to stop there: In Chapter 6, we'll show you seven more barre3 workouts to shake up your fitness routine. We've designed an 8-week plan to guide you so that you can try them all. Here's how the plan builds from week to week:

Week 1: EASING IN. During Week 1, you'll master the 10 Transformative Minutes. This standing routine is the foundation of the entire plan. It includes my most effective exercises for lifting, toning, and shaping the lower body while also burning calories and strengthening the core for improved posture. Some days, you will simply focus on doing this routine once. Other days, you will repeat it and the 5-minute Standing Stretch sequence (see page 99), building up to 30 minutes of working out. With repetition comes muscle memory—by the end of the week, you may even be able to do the workouts without referring to the book.

I'm hopeful that you're ready to fully commit to the nutrition plan from the get-go, but weaning yourself from foods that your body is accustomed to can be difficult. If you need time to ease into new ways of eating—such as drinking less coffee and more green tea, or replacing wheat flour with gluten-free alternatives—start now, with the goal of being completely committed by the end of the week. You'll learn more about how to do this in Chapter 5.

Week 2: ON BOARD. By now, you should be on board with the Love Your Lower Body nutrition plan. At the start, you may have craved some of the items you've eliminated, such as refined sugar and bread, but after just a few days without them, the hankerings have most likely tapered off. You are probably experiencing an increase of energy because your meals are fueling your body and brain with a mix of protein, healthy fats, and fiber. You'll continue to do the 10 Transformative Minutes and Standing Stretch sequence from Week 1, and you'll also learn the Full-Body Blast workout, which increases intensity by layering on targeted upper-body and core variations to the lower-body moves. You'll still have 10-minute days, but now your "long days" will include 40 minutes of activity. In this week, we introduce the idea of breaking up your longer workouts into smaller ones, starting with 10 minutes first thing in the morning. See page 128 for more about Week 2.

Week 3: DEEPEN YOUR PRACTICE. As your stamina builds, you'll find that the routines become easier, which means it's time to focus on exercises that require a higher level of mind-body awareness and detailed movements. This week, you'll learn the Love Your Lower Body Mat Workout and Mat Stretch, which require an exercise mat or a soft surface. The workout and stretch sequences use movements that are isolated, smaller, and more detailed than those in Weeks 1 and 2. These new moves will help take your practice to the next level. This week, I also introduce the core ball (and the option to use a rolled-up towel instead) to help support your body and to isolate your core and glutes. See page 156 for more about Week 3.

Week 4: MOVE ALL DAY. Researchers say that it can take up to 8 weeks to notice changes in your body due to exercise and diet, but most of our testers reported large transformations at this midpoint. To help you get there—or to boost your already remarkable results—this week is all about revving your metabolism for major calorie burn. By spreading your workouts throughout the day (rather than doing them all together), you'll increase your caloric afterburn. This week, you'll also spark your metabolism with a new workout feature to this program called a barre3 Boost. Barre3 Boosts are 1- to 5-minute full-body exercises that are designed to quickly elevate your heart rate. See page 184 for more about Week 4.

Week 5: MAKE IT YOUR OWN. By now, you have experimented with working out in one 40-minute block as well as a few 10-minute blocks throughout your day. This week, I give you a choice of two paths: working out all through the day or in one solid session. A big part of this program is tapping into your own body wisdom and learning what does and what doesn't work for you—and that includes the food you are serving up on your plate. For the past month, you have cooked a wide variety of recipes that balance protein, healthy fats, and fiber. This week, I encourage you to make your own creations, using our recipes (especially the DIY ones) and formula as your guide. See page 192 for more about Week 5.

Week 6: GET OFF YOUR BUTT. Do you know what my personal favorite benefit of barre3 is? I finally have a butt! This week kicks off with a new 10-minute Glute Combo Workout featuring Love Your Lower Body moves that will lift and shape the tush. You will do this workout in combination with your go-to Love Your Lower Body workouts from the weeks prior. You are still working out 10 minutes some days and 40 minutes others. This week, I want you to be mindful of portion sizes. You're eating the right things, but this week you'll strive to eat enough but not too much. See page 198 for more about Week 6.

Week 7: CORE VALUES. Your reflection in the mirror is transforming. Your waist is smaller, your seat is lifted, and your legs have definition. What you can't see is how your inner body is supporting all this success. This week is about working from the inside out by tapping deep into the core. We introduce a new 10-minute Love Your Lower Body Core Combo Workout made of my favorite moves that get deep into all layers of your core, including your obliques and your rectus and transverse abdominis. The core is so much more than just muscles. It is also your gut and how you digest your food. All of our recipes are designed to help clean your intestines and optimize your ability to use food as fuel to rebuild your body, burn stubborn fat, and gain mental clarity. This connection between exercise and food is at the heart of barre3's core values. See page 204 for more about Week 7.

Week 8: FULLY COMMIT. This is the most transformative week of the bunch, because it is your launchpad to living better for all the weeks to come. Consider this a fresh start rather than the end of your program. I designed this week to be memorable. It will challenge you to fully commit and trust the process, even if you haven't been giving it 100 percent thus far. This week, you will focus inward and go deep into each posture. You will give up all the foods that are not on this plan. This is going to be harder for some people than others, but I know you'll love the results! You will also have time to reflect on your goals and any surprise benefits you experienced. See page 210 for more about Week 8.

Optional: 7-DAY BODY BONUS. After the 8 weeks are over, you can continue following different combinations of the workouts you've learned to keep losing weight or maintain your loss. But if you are looking for another way to boost your burn—or a quick way to drop some extra pounds before a wedding or reunion—you can try my 7-Day Body Bonus. You will challenge yourself over this week by upping the amount of exercise you do to 60 minutes a day, 5 days a week. You will also highly focus your diet efforts to eliminate all sources of gluten and alcohol while enjoying fresh and flavorful smoothies each morning. You'll even learn a new move! See page 286 for more about the 7-Day Body Bonus.

Personalize Your Plan

The following schedule is the best way to show your lower body some love. The most crucial element to making exercise a habit is to progress at a pace that keeps you challenged and interested but not overwhelmed.

You should introduce the bonus workouts from Chapter 6 in order, but depending on your fitness level, it's okay to stay on a given week for longer than 7 days until you are ready to move on.

As for your diet, it's up to you to choose which meals you want to make and eat each day. Review the sample meal plan on page 54, or use my recipes as inspiration for your own healthy meals.

You'll be able to design and track your own workout schedule and meal plan in the journal pages in Chapter 9.

Here's a look at the number of minutes you'll be exercising each week. You can rearrange the days (swapping Day 2 and Day 3, for example), but be sure you get in all of the suggested workouts each week.

	DAY 1	DAY 2	DAY 3	DAY 4	DAY 5	DAY 6	DAY 7
WEEK 1	10 min	10 min	30 min	30 min	30 min	Rest	30 min
WEEK 2	40 min	10 min	40 min	10 min	40 min	Rest	40 min
WEEK 3	40 min	10 min	40 min	10 min	40 min	Rest	40 min
WEEK 4	40 min	10 min	40 min	10 min	40 min	Rest	40 min
WEEK 5	40 min	10 min	40 min	10 min	40 min	Rest	40 min
WEEK 6	40 min	10 min	40 min	10 min	40 min	Rest	40 min
WEEK 7	40 min	10 min	40 min	10 min	40 min	Rest	40 min
WEEK 8	40 min	10 min	40 min	10 min	40 min	Rest	40 min

Best Practices

I hope that reading about the progression of the next 2 months gets you excited and makes you confident that you'll be able to stick with it for the duration. With this plan, you don't dive right into the deep end; you slowly build strength and endurance, progressing at a healthy, effective pace. I want you to know why you're doing it and also what to expect.

There are several ways to get better results and to make this transition to healthy living easier. Before you start, here are some of my tips for success, including things I've learned on my own; from sports scientists, nutritionists, and psychologists; as well as from the 27 women who tested this plan while I was writing the book. I've divided these suggestions into two categories: (1) things you can do right now, before you start the plan, and (2) suggestions for what you can do during the next 8 weeks to make sure that as the workouts build in complexity, the plan itself becomes easier to follow.

Before You Start

Here are a few things you can do between now and your official kickoff to set yourself up for success once you're actually on the plan.

Establish a baseline. One of the tools we gave our test panelists was a preplan health assessment. On Day 1, we recorded the weight, measurements, and mood and energy levels of each woman. Every 2 weeks, we checked in with them and compared where they were at the start of the program to where they were at that moment. These women had sensed that their pants felt looser and that they had more energy in the afternoons, but seeing the results on paper gave them an extra surge of motivation.

Of course, it's up to you how you establish this baseline. If you don't want to weigh or measure yourself, you don't have to. You might find that other results are more motivating, such as how relaxed you feel at the end of the day, how easy it is to wake up in the morning, or how long you're able to hold one of the exercises without taking a break. If this is your preferred way to calculate change, I suggest you take notes about how you feel right now so you can check back on your progress.

If you want to see the numbers, I recommend using a scale that measures extra markers of health, such as percentage of body fat and pounds of lean muscle mass, but a traditional bathroom scale will do just fine. To measure the circumference of your waist, hips, legs, and arms, you'll need a tape measure. Ask a friend for help with this—otherwise, as you bend and shift to read the numbers on the tape, you can throw off the measurements.

Turn to page 298 to record your baseline measurements at the start of this program. Be sure to write in your new measurements every 2 weeks so you can track your progress.

Set goals. What is it that inspired you to pick up this book in the first place? My guess is that you have a goal or two you'd like to reach and you think this plan can help you get there. Some of the most common reasons to start a new workout and nutrition plan are:

1. To lose weight

2. To tone and shape your body

3. To increase your energy

4. To learn more about yourself and deepen your mind-body connection

Which of these describe you? Is there another reason, one that doesn't fall on this list? Whatever your answer, take a few minutes to write down why this program is important to you and how you hope it will help you achieve your goals (use the journal on page 300).

Set a few more goals. Let's set a few more goals, only this time I challenge you to have fun. Here's why: Sports scientists say that people start to exercise with a health goal in mind, such as weight loss or reducing risk of a disease like type 2 diabetes. But the reason people stick with exercise is because they are enjoying themselves in the moment. So I'm going to ask you to set extra goals for yourself, ones that will help you stay committed. If you're a social person, you might set a goal of hosting a healthy dinner party every couple of weeks so you can share your favorite recipes with friends. If you're competitive, you might challenge yourself to increase the time you can balance during poses such as Power Legs. If you're using this plan to de-stress, devote a few minutes each week to creating the cheeriest workout playlist possible. Committing to these small ways of boosting your enjoyment will ultimately pay off by making it easier to stay on track.

Go grocery shopping. You don't need any special tools for the workout portion of the Love Your Lower Body plan, but you do need specific foods for the nutrition section. I always recommend starting programs like these on a Monday so you can use the weekend to shop for ingredients and test out recipes before getting bogged down with weekday obligations. Before you begin the plan, thumb through the recipes in Chapter 7 and flag the ones that look most appealing to you. Many call for the same ingredients, and a bunch use leftovers to simplify preparation. For example, you might make Seared Tuna with Minted Quinoa Salad one night, then use the surplus to make the Tuna Niçoise Salad. Jot down a shopping list (refer to our grocery guide on page 51 for extra help), and do any extra prep work you can ahead of time, such as chopping veggies. This will minimize typical obstacles that come up when adopting a new eating plan. Keep in mind that the only things going into your shopping cart should be things you can eat on this diet: protein such as eggs, fish, beans, and nuts; healthy fats including olive oil, avocados, and coconut butter; veggies, especially dark leafy greens; fruit such as berries and apples; and whole grains like quinoa, brown rice, and whole oats.

Toss temptation. There's one foolproof way to ensure you don't succumb to cravings during the program: Make sure the unhealthy foods that usually sabotage good intentions aren't in your cabinets, fridge, or snack stash. For me, the treats I find hardest to resist are chocolate and red wine. While I preach balance and enjoy goodies from time to time, these are the things that I know need to be out of sight and reach. Red wine and chocolate rock my world in the moment but then leave me dazed and seeking the next forbidden snack. So I allow myself some on special occasions or when I go out to dinner, but the rest of the time these temptations stay out of the house, or at least remain buried at the very back of the pantry.

Cravings aside, it's smart to eliminate processed foods from your fridge and cabinets so that they're simply not an option. After a long day at the office, you may not be craving a box of macaroni and cheese, but if it's the first thing you see when you open a cabinet, there's a good chance you'll put a pot of water on to boil. On the Love Your Lower Body plan, the goal is to eat whole foods, ones that your body has an easy time recognizing. Processed foods and foods with trans fatty acids, artificial sweeteners, and artificial colors are harder for our bodies to recognize and digest. Keep whole foods handy and donate everything else to a food bank.

Recruit friends. I strongly encourage you to find friends who will join in this plan (or portions of it) with you. For me, working out and eating clean with my friends is my number one way to stay motivated and have fun along the way. We text each other to schedule times to do barre3 together or send pictures of ourselves exercising in our PJs and in silly places as we travel. We have potlucks so we can each try new recipes and share tips on how we modified them. We plan our date nights around healthy restaurants. We laugh at ourselves when we admit to cheating, and we whine once in a while about how hard substituting sparkling water is compared to drinking our favorite pinot. If you don't have immediate access to people as enthusiastic about this new way of exercising and eating as you are, you can find plenty of them in our barre3 studios and on our social media pages. From instructors to clients, there are tons of people actively sharing success stories and inspiring others to stay committed.

The benefits of getting a bit of help from your friends are backed by science. People who work out with a partner push themselves longer and harder than people who always train solo, according to a study from the University of Oxford.[1] Other research shows that friends who train together are more consistent—you're more likely to head out on a run if you know someone is waiting for you. And many studies reveal that healthy and unhealthy habits can transfer from one person to another. By surrounding yourself with healthy people, you automatically make it easier to live more healthfully yourself.

Of course, it's important to note that friends and family can support you even without following along. If none of your buddies are ready to give this program a try just yet, ask a few friends to help you stay accountable. This might mean designating a person to check in with you each day about your workouts. It might mean changing your weekly movie date with theater popcorn and candy to a night in with a rental and homemade popcorn. Tell the people in your life why this change is important. By explaining the plan to them, you'll receive fewer unhealthy invitations, and you may even inspire your friends and family to get healthier. Many of the women on my test panel found that their husbands, friends, and coworkers wanted to learn more about what they were doing after they saw one of the simple workouts or tried one of the delicious meals.

Get family support. Family can play a major role in your success. Some of the most committed barre3 students are mother-daughter duos who meet at the studio for class each morning. I have worked out with my mom my whole life. When we get together, we enjoy being active, whether that means taking walks, doing barre3, or simply splashing around a pool with my two kids in tow. Many of the recipes in this book are inspired by the ones my mom raised me on. She passed down to me a passion for eating simple, affordable, and delicious whole foods.

While my mom is aligned with this program, my husband and kids are a tougher sell. Changes in family routine can be challenging no matter what, and if the change involves major snack and mealtime makeovers, conflict might be on the horizon. It's good to go into this program knowing that you aren't going to win every battle, at least at first. If Friday night has always been pizza night, your brood may be less than thrilled to give quinoa and veggies a try. But there are ways to make the nutrition plan work without cooking separate meals each night or setting yourself up for a lot of temptation. To start, look for recipes that might appeal to the folks you need to feed. Self-assembly meals are a hit with my family of picky eaters. You can set out a bunch of different foods, like at a salad bar, for different theme nights—DIY burritos, pizzas, and omelets ensure everyone can make healthy choices they enjoy.

The same goes for exercise. Chances are at least some of your workouts will be done at home, and if you have an audience of curious kiddos or a confused partner, spend a little time instructing them through the moves.

They'll learn that the workouts aren't nearly as easy as they look, and you might even get them to join you. When my daughter sees me doing Standing Leg Lifts (page 152) in the kitchen, she often follows along. Jennifer Dashney-Longbine, one of the test panelists, had her toddler twins shadowing her for almost every workout. It's even become a game for a lot of my clients: They post photos on Facebook of unexpected family members catching the barre3 wave at home. There are dads in Ohio doing it, moms with triplets, and everyone's favorite—babies who make their own way into plank pose!

Avoid the shame spiral. This tip really belongs in the "As You Progress" section on page 77, but I want to bring up the topic now—before you start the plan. One thing that was often mentioned by the test panel was an overwhelming sense of guilt when someone cheated. Maybe she missed a day of working out, maybe she had half of a cookie at an office party. These "cheats" were usually small infractions, although sometimes there were much larger slipups. The fact is, these things happen. They happened to our panelists, they've happened to me, and they're going to happen to you. We all have moments of weakness, or of feeling overwhelmed, or of just plain forgetting what we've committed to on this plan. The important thing is not to beat yourself up about it. All you can do is accept the mistake and move on.

About halfway through the 8 weeks, one of the panelists said she'd had a day where she'd not only fallen off the wagon but had, in her words, "smashed the wagon." Her back hurt enough from a prior injury that she missed her morning workouts. This brought on a wave of guilt so strong that she binged at breakfast, eating pastries, bacon, and all sorts of other foods she'd been shying away from. She topped it off with a cup of coffee. If she was feeling bad before, she felt downright awful afterward.

A simple slipup, like missing a workout, can lead to feelings of self-loathing that blow the mistake out of proportion and cause even more interruptions. Your confidence plummets, the guilt sets in, and you make choices that are often much poorer and larger than the initial misdeed. It's as if you actually want to prove that you have zero willpower, or that you're destined to fail, or that you can't do anything right.

One of the best approaches I have learned over the years to combat this negative spiral is to take a deep breath and simply observe my behavior and how I feel rather than beating myself up for it. It might be as simple as saying, "I'm eating ice cream, and I feel bad about it." I find that being honest with myself—without judgment—relieves pressure. With less pressure on ourselves, we are more likely to make good choices and shrug off the bad ones. Try it!

Robyn Conley Downs, a client who has been following the barre3 workout and eating philosophy for more than a year, shared this story that helps put things in perspective. Hopefully, you'll remember her words when you find yourself starting to go down this dark road.

I am part of the most amazing book club. We are 12 women who get together every month to socialize and really talk about the book. These ladies take the discussion very seriously. They also take wine and cheese very seriously. I'm telling you this because we met last night, and as usual there was a full spread of delicious-looking cheese, desserts, and plenty of wine. I didn't bring my own food because I just didn't feel like it, but I did eat a good dinner before I went.

I settled in for the evening with my ice water and didn't think twice about bypassing the wine and cheese. But then the host served just-out-of-the-oven homemade brownies. I bypassed those for about an hour or so, too. But then I decided I really, really wanted one. So I ate one. Actually, I ate one and a half, if I'm being honest. And I didn't eat them with protein or fiber or anything to stabilize my blood sugar.

In the past, I would have thought of this as cheating, and it may have led me to thinking I'd fallen off the wagon. And one brownie might have led to a what-the-heck-why-not weekend of lousy eating choices.

But I don't think that way anymore. Instead, I just enjoyed a really good brownie with my friends. I considered it a special treat. And I got up today and had my smoothie and worked out really hard. I think I sweated the brownie out, if that's possible. And I ate kale for dinner, with protein, which definitely balanced out the brownies. It's nice to know that a few treats here or there are not going to ruin everything. Just enjoy it and get back to the program.

Cheers to that!

As You Progress

Once you're following the Love Your Lower Body plan, these suggestions can help you stay focused, motivated, and safe, all while improving your results.

Journal your progress. Health experts are all in agreement about this one: When you write down what you eat and how much you exercise, you automatically improve your health habits. Putting your actions on paper helps you avoid negative behaviors and improves your adherence to more positive changes. You'll be less likely to grab a cookie in a staff meeting if you know you must record it in your food log, and you'll be more inspired to fit in your workouts if you get to check them off of your to-do list. In fact, a study in the *American Journal of Preventive Medicine* found that dieters who kept a food diary lost twice as much weight as dieters who didn't.[2] That's a lot of extra pounds lost for not a whole lot of extra effort.

To help you out, Chapter 9 offers an 8-week journal for you to fill in as you progress through the plan. There's space for you to record your nutrition and exercise for each day. There's also room for you to make notes about your successes. You might want to indicate such milestones as the first day you were able to do an entire 10-minute routine without taking a break. Or you might put stars next to the recipes you love and want to repeat. Be sure to record the nonphysical changes, too. Noting nights when you slept particularly well or challenging days that didn't boost your stress levels can help you stay excited about all the changes you're experiencing.

Of course, there are lots of ways to record your transformation. If pen and paper don't appeal to you, maybe you'd rather share your successes via social media or start a blog about your journey. Although this is an optional part of the plan, keeping some record of your daily actions and feelings is a proven way to get better results.

Listen to your body. The goal of this program is to help you feel stronger and more confident, but that doesn't mean you're going to roll out of bed with energy to spare each morning. On some days, particularly in the beginning, you may find that you're tired or that your muscles are sore from this new routine. That's why the workout schedule is a suggestion, not a set plan to follow. If 40 minutes of exercise on Monday leaves you feeling drained on Tuesday morning, then Tuesday might be a day to go easier on yourself with a single 10-minute workout. Conversely, if one morning you wake up refreshed before your alarm clock rings, you might elect to sneak in 20 minutes of fitness before your shower. I find that I get the best results when I plan my days in advance, then allow for in-the-moment changes based on how I'm feeling physically and mentally.

It's important to listen to your body. Each time you move through a workout, keep assessing and reassessing how you feel. For instance, if your shoulders are aching or you woke up with a crick in your neck, you might want to hold your arms at shoulder height or lower during the upper-body exercises or ditch the handheld weights. Each day will be different, so don't ignore physical or emotional cues; whether you're full of vigor or feeling a little overworked, there's a way to make this plan fit your body and your mood. The goal is to balance your sense of ease and effort in each of the exercises. I find that giving yourself permission to find the ease is actually the most challenging part.

One of the test panelists who tried this plan, Megan Schendel, had this to say about taking it day by day: "I've noticed that my body is ready for a bigger challenge on some days and less of a challenge on others. I have chronic knee pain, so I spread my workouts out to give my muscles and joints a rest. When I'm feeling good, I focus on getting lower in the postures, doing slow and deliberate movements, and really making sure I'm completely engaged. I also do a couple of workouts back-to-back to intensify the experience."

Look for things you like. I know that following this plan won't always be easy. That's why it's important to focus on all of the ways your life is improving.

Take test panelist Angie Thomason, for example. At the start of the program, she was most excited about losing weight—her original goal was to lose 2 pounds a week. But as time went on, what she really looked forward to was the way she felt after doing the workouts. "If I had a stressful day, the workouts actually helped me erase all of that tension," said Thomason.

TAKE A SELFIE

Before you get started on the diet and exercise plan, take a few "before" pics. As you track your changes on the scale and in your measurements, it can be nice to see how these losses affect your appearance. One of my regular clients, Annie Eeds, has lost more than 75 pounds by following my barre3 workout and diet plan, and she told me that she is addicted to taking "after" photos every few weeks and comparing them to the befores. For her, it is a way to literally see her progress and to be proud of how far she has come. She told me that the pictures tell her so much more than the scale, which is just a number that can go up and down. These super-quick self-portraits capture just how happy, fit, and balanced she is. (To read her story, turn to page 338.)

"I noticed that the scale didn't matter as much. Instead, I was excited to see how my body was changing, but I mainly focused on how I felt."

Panelist Jennifer Dashney-Longbine had a totally different approach. She started making power-packed playlists for her workouts, then used the music to keep herself motivated and challenged. "Moving to the beat made me feel like I was dancing, not exercising," she explained. "Plus, I sang along with my playlists, which made the routine feel more like fun and less like work."

The reasons you ultimately stick with the Love Your Lower Body plan will be unique to you. Maybe you find that exercising for 10 minutes each morning keeps you more focused at work, or that by exercising in front of your husband he's more likely to exercise, too. You may realize that you love the taste of kale and almond butter. Whatever little joys you find in the workout and diet plan—from your in-the-moment experience to how you feel afterward—use these mini-victories to stay inspired.

Don't dwell on disappointment. There will be days when the number on the scale doesn't budge or you're feeling stressed despite all of your good intentions. This is normal! Big, life-lasting change takes time, so don't get discouraged. Focus on the positives and try to look past any negatives. Think about how your clothes are fitting, or how much firmer your body appears, or how much extra energy you have in the afternoon. Trust me on this: If you keep doing the work, you are going to have success.

Go for extra credit. The suggested schedules I created for each week of the plan highlight the minimum amount of exercise I'd like you to get, but if you're inspired to do more, go for it! After tackling a 10-minute routine, I sometimes get inspired to stay active, even if it's nothing more than a spontaneous dance party with my 8- and 9-year-old kids. This is when I know my program is working—when I make choices after my workouts that still support my goals. Every moment of exercise will bring you closer, helping you burn calories and build strength and endurance. But don't overdo it. Remember to listen to your body so that you avoid feeling depleted. Pushing your body past its limits can set you up for injury or burnout, which can sabotage your success.

Reward yourself. It's easy to focus on a big goal and forget to celebrate the smaller successes. But by rewarding yourself all along the way, you'll stay more motivated throughout your journey. Jot down a few milestones you're looking forward to, such as losing your first 5 pounds or finishing a workout without taking a break. When you attain one, treat yourself. You might schedule a pedicure, go shopping for a new workout top, or simply set aside an entire hour to read. Choose a gift that's in line with your goals: Cupcakes are out, a new workout headband is in.

Raising the Barre

ALEX NOWLIN

AGE: 34　　　**POUNDS LOST:** 7.8　　　**INCHES LOST:** $7\frac{3}{4}$ *including $3\frac{1}{2}$ from her waist and 2 from her hips*

I have historically been a healthy, athletic person, but after my pregnancy, my muscle tone and physical shape were not the same. My son, Drake, who was born 8 months before the Love Your Lower Body test panel started, was breech, and I had a mandatory C-section. I think a lot of women can relate to the state of your abdominal muscles post–C-section—they're practically nonexistent. On top of that, I work full-time, and my husband spends much of his time on the road for his job. I signed up for the test panel because I wanted to "lose the baby weight" and rehabilitate from my pregnancy, but I was also hoping I'd find more balance and energy along the way.

Right from the start, I was amazed at how effective a 10-minute workout could be. I had thought I needed 20 to 30 minutes of cardio to be effective, and that your heart rate should be elevated for a certain duration, which was nearly impossible with a young child around.

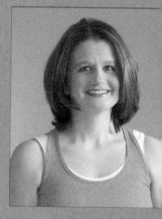

Even on the barre3 plan, there were times that I couldn't get a full 10 minutes in without interruption. I would do a few minutes, pick the baby up, then finish later. Or I would hold him while doing the moves. I didn't have time to change into workout clothes, but it didn't matter. This flexibility allowed me to get the exercise in, even if it wasn't perfect.

Thanks to the diet, there are a lot of foods that I am no longer tempted by. I will never view sugar the same again. My body feels so much better now that I'm cautious about my sugar intake. In the past, I never felt satisfied after having just fruit for a snack. I now realize that my blood sugar is extremely sensitive to sugar. Adding protein to meals and snacks was a huge part of my success and allowed me to sustain energy throughout the day. When I do have something sweet, it is because I truly want it, and it better be good. The plan really helped me clean up my act and focus more on the food choices I was making through the day.

Eight weeks in, I am in much better physical shape and my whole family is eating differently, even the little guy. When I mentioned to my husband that it looked like he'd lost weight, his response was, "It's because of your diet." Following the plan for 8-plus weeks has helped me to develop habits that are now part of my daily routine.

I LOVE MY LOWER BODY *because:*

I love the strength that I have in my lower body, which supports the rest of my body all day long. I notice the muscle strength I have in class, when doing other sports like jogging or hiking, or simply running errands around town.

Chapter 5

Week 1:
The 10
Transformative
MINUTES

IT'S TIME TO MOVE! DURING WEEK 1 OF THIS PLAN, YOU'LL LEARN AND master my cornerstone workout, the 10 Transformative Minutes. This workout has it all. The poses shape your calves, your quads, your hamstrings, your glutes, and your abs—basically everything below your rib cage. You'll get your heart rate up, wear your muscles out, and burn major calories, all in just 10 minutes a pop. You'll ease into the program by doing the routine once a day. By the end of the week, you'll be doing two rounds of the workout each day plus a stretch sequence that will help your body recover and reset. This first week, you're going to work on perfecting the 10 Transformative Minutes. After that, you'll start to add new moves and workouts, most of which build on this basic routine. That's why it's so important you work to get it right this week. It truly is the foundation of the next 8 weeks.

Starting Week 1

The habits you begin to establish during these first few days of the eating program will last for the next 8 weeks. If you haven't already, look ahead to the recipes in Chapter 7 and select a few to try. Pick a couple of different breakfasts, lunches, snacks, and dinners and strive to have all of the necessary groceries on hand. I suggest you do as much prep work ahead of time as possible—cutting veggies, cooking quinoa—to make mealtimes smooth and seamless. I often cook in large batches so I have leftovers to eat and to transform into other meals. I might make tacos one night, then eat the surplus chicken and veggies as a bowl for lunch the next day. Try to map out your meals ahead of time so you're never stuck without something healthy to eat. Of course, you can't plan for every contingency, so be sure to have several of the grab-and-go snacks available, just in case.

Which recipes you choose this week and every week are completely up to you. At the start, I suggest you pick ones with ingredients you already know you like—then try some of the more adventurous dishes later in the program. All of the foods in these recipes and on the shopping list will help your body get a nutritious balance of protein, healthy fats, and fiber. These foods will maintain your energy for your workouts and for your whole day. As you become increasingly familiar with pairing foods for optimum flavor and nutrition, you can experiment on your own, using the recipes and grocery list as a starting place.

Here are some hints to help you get the most out of this first week.

Ease In for Results

One guiding principle of this whole program is to balance ease and effort. For the workouts, your goal is to figure out how to make each posture feel good in your body while making it challenging. I find that most of us err on the challenging side when starting a new program. We jump all the way in and attempt to do everything fast and furiously—and then end up burning out. When starting a new routine, finding ease can be a challenge. The same applies to the nutrition program. It's tempting to try new recipes for each meal each day, but for most of us, this isn't sustainable. Cost, time spent in the kitchen, and wasted leftovers all add up. To make the most of your effort, you might want to double recipes so you have plenty of leftovers. Or pick one meal a day to phase in this new style of eating.

Get Familiar with the Workout

These are 10-minute workouts, but you might want to give yourself a full half hour for your first run-through. Each exercise comes with thoroughly detailed instructions, including how your body should be positioned from heels to head, where your weight should be, and how to move in the position. Focus on your placement initially—I want you to move only after you're safely set up. You may find that it helps to have a large mirror nearby to ensure your knees really are over your ankles and your shoulders really are in line with your hips. By the end of the week, you won't need a mirror, because you'll know what good alignment feels like.

TOOLS TO TRY

Some of the exercises in the Love Your Lower Body workouts can be done standing in the center of the room, no props required. Others may call for a couple of simple items, most of which you may already own. Here are the tools I use on this plan.

Ballet Barre

Barre3 studios have a wall-mounted ballet barre to help clients align and stabilize, but you don't need a ballet barre to do these workouts. All you need is a waist-high surface such as the back of a kitchen chair. Some exercises require a sturdier surface, such as a kitchen counter or the back of a heavy couch.

Exercise Mat

Some of the exercises require getting on the floor. A yoga mat can provide a bit of padding between you and the ground. You'll want a mat starting in Week 3.

Light Handheld Weights

You don't need weights to tone your arms, but we do suggest them as an option in some of our combination workouts starting in Week 2. At my studios, we supply 1- to 3-pound handheld weights; most of my clients use 2-pounders.

Core Ball

We use the core ball to help you get deep into the core, inner thighs, seat, and more. This ball is a great travel companion—it's easy to inflate (no pump required) and easy to pack; the 9-inch ball has more give to it than a typical toy ball. (You can purchase a core ball online at shop.barre3.com.) If you don't have the ball handy, use a rolled-up towel. Simply fold a standard hotel-size towel in half lengthwise, then roll it up and use it in place of the ball. We'll start using this tool during Week 3.

MOVE WITH INTENTION

These Love Your Lower Body workouts are a time to check in, not check out. If you pay attention to how your body feels and how it's moving through space, you'll be tuned in to any adjustments you need to make, ultimately giving yourself a better workout. If your muscles aren't starting to enter that burning phase after a minute or so, you may need to use the "get deeper" instructions I have outlined for you. If your muscles are on fire the moment you start to move, it may be an indication to ease up a little and focus on breathing. This self-focus will improve your exercise session so that it may even feel like an active meditation: By training yourself to spend more time reflecting on how you feel, you become more attuned to the other benefits of working out, such as extra energy or a mood boost. Also, by focusing on the detail of movement, you'll be living in the moment, making it harder for your to-do list and other daily stressors to creep into your thoughts.

Also, be sure to try out the modifications to see if different ways of doing an exercise feel better on your body. These small variations are designed to help you work deeply even if you have limitations such as back or knee problems. At first, April Abernethy, one of my test panelists, resisted modifying. "I'm a former gymnast, so taking the 'easier' option made me feel like I was a quitter," said Abernethy. "But now I modify all the time. I've realized that these changes help me work just as deeply, if not more so." Panelist Frayn Masters had the same experience: "As a former athlete, I had to get used to the idea that modifications are not cheating, are not inferior. But some days, I feel so strong and powerful I can go deep, deep, deep, and other days my hip flexors are screaming at me and I modify. I finally learned that no one else cares whether I'm modifying or not. As long as I am taking care of myself, finding new ways to go deeper, finding new focus and staying the course—that is what matters." In a typical barre3 studio class, you would see clients using a wide array of modifications during a single exercise. The more you do these moves, the more I encourage you to modify and make them your own.

Get Familiar with the Food

I love reading cookbooks: looking at the ingredient lists and instructions, and taking note of the ones I'm looking forward to trying. I encourage you to read some of the recipes just as you would any other portion of the book. Become familiar with the types of foods you'll be eating and how they're combined for optimal nutrition. It's also a good idea to make a copy or take a picture of the grocery list in Chapter 3. Refer to this frequently to help you get a handle on what to eat when you don't have the full nutrition plan in front of you, such as when you're shopping, dining out, or traveling.

Plan Your Workouts

You've probably heard that scheduling your workouts can help you fit them in your day, and it's no different on this program. I find that I like to do at least one 10-minute Love Your Lower Body workout first thing each morning—before I start to fall behind on my to-do list, which can make it

DRESS FOR SUCCESS

There is no official dress code for these workouts—feel free to wear anything that allows you to move without restriction. I regularly exercise in yoga attire, pajamas, and even street clothes—it depends on what I'm doing when the urge to move strikes!

When possible, I recommend doing this workout in bare feet. Going barefoot can stabilize and strengthen the muscles of the feet and improve your balance and overall performance. However, the moves are easily doable in sneakers and socks—which I recommend if you need extra support and cushioning.

SOOTHE SORE MUSCLES

All of this extra movement might make for sore and tired muscles. Here are three of my favorite ways to reward my body for all the hard work it does.

- **A SOAK IN THE TUB**: Add 2 cups of Epsom salts and a few drops of lavender essential oil to your bath. Lavender is an effective aromatherapy cure for stress, and Epsom salts release lactic acid buildup in your muscles.

- **ACUPUNCTURE**: I recently told my acupuncturist, Sarah Hayes, that going to her was like instant Savasana—the feeling you get during Corpse Pose in yoga class when your mind is clear and your body is relaxed. I went in for my first session scared of needles and left feeling like I had just spent hours at a spa. Now I crave those tiny needles!

- **A FANCY PEDICURE**: My husband recently splurged and bought me a pedicure at a day spa. It was a totally different experience than the express pedis I usually get. It included an exfoliation, a paraffin dip, and a great foot and calf massage. You're looking at your toes a lot during these 8 weeks—treat them well!

tempting to skip exercise. The women who tested this plan had a number of different strategies when it came to fitting in multiple workouts in a day. Some would plan workouts for right before or after mealtime. (You read about the benefits of both of these strategies in Chapter 2.) Others saved the 10-minute routines for times they needed more energy, such as midafternoon or right after work. Still others grouped the workouts into 20- and 30-minute chunks and did longer back-to-back toning sessions, which can feel more challenging than shorter, separate sessions. All of these options—and more—are available to you, so test-drive a few ways of working. Just be sure you start each day with a game plan so that you don't push your workouts off and into the next day.

Plan Your Meals

Here's a moment you want to avoid on this plan: wandering into the kitchen, opening the fridge, and rooting around to find something to eat. These aimless moments are the times you're most likely to veer off track, so be sure you have the right groceries on hand for a few grab-and-go snacks if not full-blown meals. I always have hummus and chopped veggies in the fridge and Chocolate-Hazelnut Bites (page 283) in the freezer. Because fresh produce is best the day of purchase or up to 2 days after, I do tend to make at least a couple of quick trips to the store each week. Pick a few breakfast and dinner recipes to shop for, then think about ways to turn the leftovers into snacks and lunches. With a bit of extra quinoa and kale, you can make last night's dinner tomorrow's new-and-improved lunch.

Create Healthy Habits

Part of the reason you're doing the same workout multiple times this week is to perfect your form and your movements and commit them to memory. Don't worry that this plan will be too simple or boring this week. I've found that doing the same exact exercises over and over again actually makes the moves more challenging over time, not easier. Why is this? There are dozens of ways to get deeper into each movement just by making small adjustments to your form. The best challenge for your body and your brain is repetition, not new choreography.

I know it can be tempting to skim the instructions or flip ahead in the book, but it's crucial that you focus on and embrace these core exercises before moving on. If you take the time to learn and master these movements, you will build a strong foundation and a clear understanding of what these Love Your Lower Body routines are supposed to feel like. This will help you reach your goals for the entire 8 weeks and beyond.

The same is true with the eating plan. As you try out some of these recipes, I encourage you to repeat your favorites. Unfamiliarity is much of the reason a new diet might feel challenging at first. Each time you make a dish, you'll shave off minutes because you'll have learned shortcuts or memorized steps. After just a few tries, these new meals will be as easy to fix as some of your tried-and-true recipes.

Go Deeper with Your Workouts

The first several run-throughs of the 10 Transformative Minutes may pose a real challenge to your body. You may experience fatigued-muscle shakes and quakes almost as soon as you start each exercise, which is a sure sign you're pushing yourself to your limit. But in less time than you might think, your body will understand the effort it takes to do these exercises. By the end of this first week, the routine might start to feel a little, well, easy. That's when it's time to learn to work deeper into each move.

One of the things I love the most about barre3 is that it gets harder the longer you do it. The better you know your body, the more quickly you can move straight to that quaking and shaking zone where your muscles are working to the max. I include suggestions to "get deeper" in each exercise write-up, but here are some of the most common ways to get the most out of each exercise.

- **Find your feet.** Your feet are your foundation, but they rarely get attention in traditional fitness. I've found that by rooting all four corners of your feet to the floor during certain moves, you can target the muscles in the backs of your legs. By gripping the floor with the base of your toes in other poses, you'll activate your inner thighs. Paying attention to how your feet connect to the floor can change the way you do the exercise. When I cue you to root evenly through all four corners of your feet in certain poses, my goal is to help you avoid putting your weight on the outer or inner edges of your feet. Aim to spread your weight evenly on the corners of each foot while keeping an active arch in the center. Avoid pressing your whole foot flat to the ground. (You can think of a tree with its roots pressing into the earth and providing balance and stability.)

- **Use your imagination.** Some of my favorite cues are telling people to find more resistance by harnessing the power of their thoughts. Here's what I mean: You might be doing biceps curls without a

THE POWER OF THE INCH

Moving big can lift your heart rate, but it also gives your muscles time to rest at the top and bottom of the movement. By moving your body just 1 inch, your muscles stay contracted the entire time so you reach that place of fatigue faster. Here are some things to remember when you're moving just 1 inch.

HOLD BEFORE MOVING. In each posture, you will stay in alignment and hold for five deep breaths before moving. You are holding in your challenge zone before you take your small 1-inch movements.

1 INCH IS SMALL. This small movement is hard! That's why it's easy for 1 inch to quickly turn into 3 or 4 inches. Don't let this happen. I want your movements to be barely perceptible. You are just 1 inch away from standing completely still.

1 INCH IS SLOW. For some reason, a lot of people equate small movements with speed. But your muscles have to work harder when you take momentum out of the exercise. Like an inhale and exhale, moving both down and up are important. Slow it down and the results will come even faster.

1 INCH IS CONTROLLED. When you're moving just 1 inch, your body shouldn't look like it's bouncing in a saddle. Work to move at a steady, slow, and controlled pace.

KEEP BREATHING. With 1 inch, you are moving small but breathing big. You might find yourself taking small, shallow breaths. Focus instead on taking full, deep inhales and exhales.

weight, but if you imagine that you're holding a heavy weight and focus on resisting this weight as you pull it in and push it away, you're going to work your biceps more than you would otherwise.

• **Focus inward.** In Pilates classes, you'll often hear instructors encourage students to hug or draw their muscles in toward an imaginary center line that divides the body lengthwise. I suggest the same thing in barre3. Hugging your muscles inward and toward this imaginary line trains your body to work the deep core muscles, creating stability and a strong foundation for developing a long, lean physique.

- **Play with depth.** Almost all of the standing moves in this book involve a knee bend; the deeper you go, the harder your muscles have to work. But this isn't a call to squat with your hips dropped down so they touch your ankles. The place where your muscles have the most strength is midcontraction—or when your knees are partially, but not fully, bent. If you find your muscles aren't firing much, you may want to bend your knees a little deeper. If your knees are achy, you can come up a little higher so that you work above any feelings of pain or tenderness.

- **Harness your core strength.** Many of the moves in the Love Your Lower Body plan are leg exercises, but that doesn't mean the rest of your body should be relaxed. Your core, in particular, plays an important role in this fitness program, regardless of whether you're standing, squatting, or lying down. By engaging your abdominal muscles for the duration of each workout, you'll better maintain good form and also move with more control, which can help you work harder and burn more calories. At first, you might find that tapping into your core strength isn't as easy as you'd expect. That's why I've included detailed cues with each exercise description to remind you how to work from the inside out.

- **Focus on intervals.** As you do the workouts, notice how you can increase and decrease your heart rate by pushing your muscles to failure, then taking an active recovery. Varying periods of work and rest during exercise is called interval training, and it's an extremely efficient way to get in a workout. The Love Your Lower Body routines are sequenced to be interval training. You first hold postures and then layer on small movements to slightly elevate the heart rate. Next, you layer on dynamic movement that quickly raises the heart rate. After about a minute, you return to a hold or transition into a stretch to bring the heart rate back down. This cycle revs your metabolism and works efficiently to

SHAKES AND QUAKES

There's one easy way to tell if you're pushing yourself to your limits during your Love Your Lower Body workouts: Your muscles start shaking uncontrollably. We call that sensation "barre3 earthquakes," and it's a good indication that you've truly fatigued your muscles, especially the larger ones like your quads and hamstrings. These alpha muscles, also called fast-twitch muscles, burn out pretty fast during isometric holds and small movements. As they fatigue, the stabilizer muscles, also known as slow-twitch muscles, start to take over. The shaking comes from these stabilizers fighting to keep you upright. Shaking and quaking is a good thing—it means you're getting stronger. Activating the stabilizer muscles is key to sculpting long, lean lines rather than bulk, which can occur when you focus only on the major muscle groups.

You may notice that during the first week of following this plan, you shake and quake during each workout. As you get stronger, that feeling may not come so automatically. That's why I've included many suggestions for how to work deeper on each exercise. Athletes get right into these shakes because they know how to recruit and tax these muscles from the get-go. When you learn how to do this, the workout naturally gets harder because you're pushing your edge and working at your max. The faster you get to the limit-pushing part of a pose, the faster you're going to burn those muscles out.

If you're not getting the quakes and shakes with each workout, it means you can go deeper. That's where the mind-body connection comes in. If you're present, if you're focused on your workout, you will have an easier time getting your muscles to fire. Stay aware of what your body is doing at all times and play around with ways to engage your muscles more, from changing the placement of your feet to using your imagination to help you create resistance. (You'll learn more about working deeper in Chapter 6.) Once you have a handle on the sequences, it's up to you to find ways to get even more out of each exercise.

PRIMARY POSTURE:
TRAIN YOUR BODY TALL

n barre3, the most important posture is primary posture. When you stand tall in this position, your body is optimally aligned. Your ligaments and muscles support the joints to prevent the risk of injury, and your spine is in neutral position, where your back has natural curves. Your feet are weighted evenly, and the muscles of your front, back, and sides are working equally. Your whole body works better when you're in this balanced, fully upright position. You breathe better, digest your food better, and minimize the potential for aches and pains.

Each exercise in this program works strategically to help balance your body so that standing in primary posture is effortless. Many of the barre3 postures work with a long spine in neutral to reinforce this alignment. Other postures that move the spine out of neutral alignment, such as rolls that move between rounding and extending the spine, work to open up tight areas of the body and strengthen weak areas so you can stand tall with ease.

In primary posture, your shoulders are wide and down your back and stacked over your hips. Your knees are soft, and your feet are hip-width apart and facing forward. This is the alignment I want you to come back to when you need to rest during exercise.

By resetting your body in primary posture, your shoulders will relax, your back with lengthen, and your core will engage. As this position grows more familiar, try standing in it throughout the day. Ideally, this posture will become the natural way you carry your body—not just while exercising, but all day long.

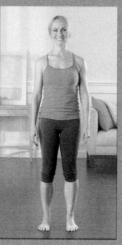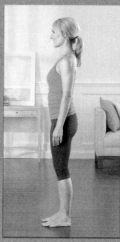

tone your body. To make the most of these changes in training intensity, focus on using the methods I've described to get deeper even more quickly. The faster you get to that place of pushing your limits, the more effective your intervals will be.

- **Tune in, not out.** It's tempting to try to multitask, talking on the phone or making a mental to-do list while getting in your reps. But by truly focusing on your movements, you'll be able to work at your full potential, getting the most out of every inch and breath as you shape your body and de-stress your mind. This is particularly important at the beginning of the plan, when you're still learning the moves, figuring out how to activate certain muscles, and working to keep your breath and your balance. But even when you get the hang of the movements, exercising without distraction can ensure you're giving each workout your all, not just going through the motions.

Test panelist Frayn Masters said that during the times when she was most focused on her movements was when she really began to understand them. "It was when I was focused that both the micro- and macro-victories occurred," said Masters. "It was when I was concentrating that I was able to figure out how to engage my muscles and connect them for movement—I would have an aha moment of sorts, and a little bit of elation. I would go from feeling like I was lugging my body through an exercise to being able to go deeper, experience exactly how my body works, and connect into my full strength."

Don't Skip the Stretch

I've created the 5-minute Love Your Lower Body Standing Stretch to bring length and relief to the muscles you work during the 10 Transformative Minutes. Stretching can help the body recover from hard work, and it can also improve your flexibility. I've seen clients who add stretching to their workouts get to the point where they can finally touch their toes, which is a huge victory. The more mobile you are, the easier everyday life will become. Stretching can help you do all sorts of tasks, from lifting bags into an overhead compartment to improving your running stride.

10 Transformative Minutes

This initial short routine doesn't require any fancy props or fitness attire. When I first started doing this workout, I treated it like a typical fitness routine, putting on workout clothes and finding a quiet, private space. But over time, I learned all of that was unnecessary. Now I do this workout whenever the urge hits, even if I'm still in my street clothes, regardless of whether I'm in my office, at an airport, in the park, or in my kitchen. This workout is something you integrate into your life, no matter where you live or what you do for a living.

CHEAT SHEET

Each exercise includes simple instructions, detailing how to move in a pose and for how long. Below is a guide to reading these shorthand notes.

RANGE: The size of your movement.

● **Hold**: Get into a position and stay there without moving.

● **1 inch**: Move in a small 1-inch range of motion while keeping your muscles engaged. For example: In Horse Pose with Heels Lifted, you will find your starting position, then lower your hips 1 inch, then lift them 1 inch.

● **Large**: Move bigger while keeping your muscles engaged. For example: In Horse Pose Pliés, you will find your starting position, then use your legs to fully stand before lowering back down.

REPS: The number of times you'll do each movement.

TIME: The amount of time it will take you to complete the repetitions.

These moves are the ones you would do in almost every barre3 studio workout. They are wildly popular because they quickly shape your body, improve your strength and endurance, and give you long-term postural benefits. The exercises work opposing muscle groups to bring balance and proportion to your body. For example, the Power Leg exercise heats and strengthens the fronts of your thighs, while Sumo Squats strengthen your hamstrings and glutes to lift and shape the backside of your body.

Although the focus of these moves is on toning the lower body, these exercises also reinforce a graceful upright posture. The instruction for each exercise includes cues to engage your core, lengthen your spine, and open your chest, all of which contribute to good alignment. Because these exercises work multiple muscles at once and are challenging enough to fatigue your body quickly, this routine is incredibly time efficient. Ten minutes isn't a lot of time, so I've made every second count.

This Week's Schedule

This workout strengthens and tones all of the muscles in the lower body and core. To make it a true 10-minute workout, limit your rest time between moves, particularly as your endurance increases. By moving straight from one pose to the next, you'll keep your heart rate up and ensure you get in the maximum benefit from each workout. On the coming pages, you will find the workout at a glance. You'll notice that in the first days, you'll do the 10 Transformative Minutes once a day, building throughout the week to doing it twice daily with the 5-minute Standing Stretch sequence, which you will also learn in this chapter. If you are starting this program having not exercised for several months, feel free to take an extra week to build up your endurance and really learn these moves. It's essential to pay close attention to your posture, which you can do by practicing in front of a mirror at first. Once you are comfortable with the 10 Transformative Minutes, you'll be able to move on with the rest of the 8-week plan. Turn the page to learn each movement in detail.

Week 1

DAY 1	DAY 2	DAY 3	DAY 4	DAY 5	DAY 6	DAY 7
10 min	10 min	30 min	30 min	30 min	Rest	30 min

On Days 1 and 2, you will do the 10 Transformative Minutes.

On Days 3, 4, 5, and 7, you will do the 10 Transformative Minutes and the Standing Stretch twice.

Days 3, 4, 5 & 7

10 Transformative Minutes

New!

Horse Pose Pliés p.100

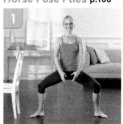

Horse Pose with Heels Lifted p.102

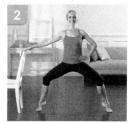

Starfish p.104

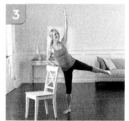

Carousel Horse p.106

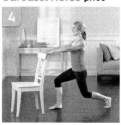

Narrow Athletic V p.108

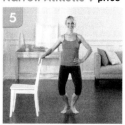

Narrow Athletic V Twists p.110

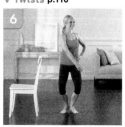

Sumo Squats p.112

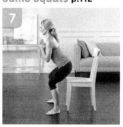

Power Leg p.114

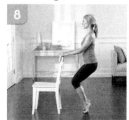

Standing Leg Lift p.116

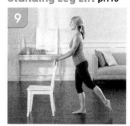

Plank p.118

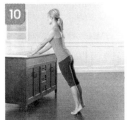

Standing Stretch

New!

Triceps Foldover p.120

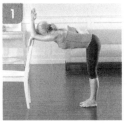

IT Band Stretch with a Twist p.121

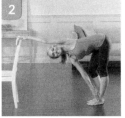

Crescent Lunge with Chest Opener p.122

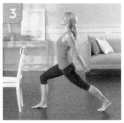

Heel to Seat Stretch p.123

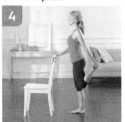

Figure 4 p.124

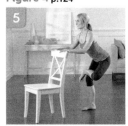

Horse Pose Pliés

SETUP: Come to Horse Pose by stepping out wider than your hips with your feet turned out to 2 and 10 o'clock. Your shoulders are stacked over your hips and your core is engaged. Bend your knees and slide your back 6 inches down an imaginary wall. Your knees are over your ankles and in line with your second toes. Your arms are low. Hold for 5 deep breaths.

MOVEMENT 1: Push down with your feet and straighten your legs. At the same time, sweep your arms to the sides and above your head.

MOVEMENT 2: Bend your knees and lower 6 inches. Sweep your arms down.

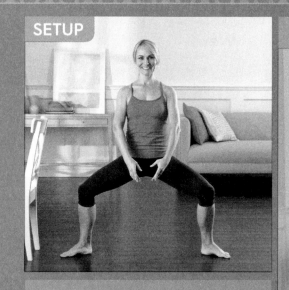

SETUP

1

We call this posture Horse Pose because it reminds me of horseback riding. Just like riding a horse, this pose works your legs as well as your postural muscles to help you find grace and ease in your stance.

GET DEEPER:

- Engage your core.
- Root all four corners of your feet evenly to the floor.
- Hug in your inner thighs as if you were riding a horse.
- Relax your shoulders down your back.

MODIFICATION:

- To minimize knee or hip discomfort, work higher or move your feet into a narrower stance.

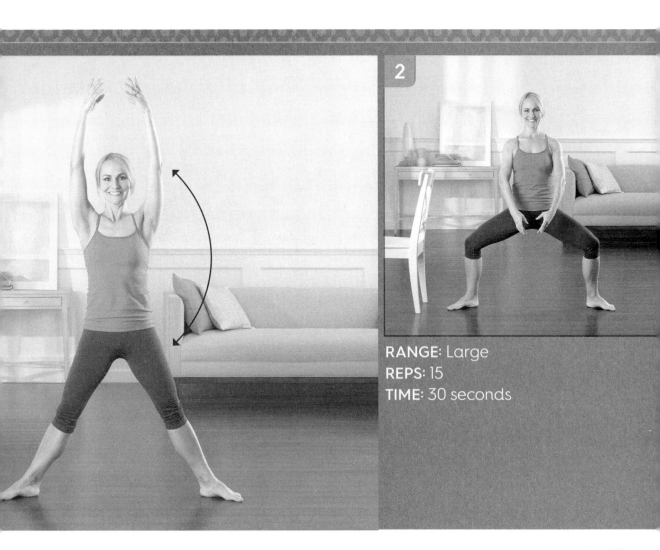

RANGE: Large
REPS: 15
TIME: 30 seconds

Horse Pose with Heels Lifted

SETUP: Stand in profile with your right hip next to the barre. Come to Horse Pose by stepping out wider than your hips with your feet turned out to 2 and 10 o'clock. Your shoulders are stacked over your hips and your core is engaged. Bend your knees and slide your back 6 inches down an imaginary wall. Your knees are over your ankles and in line with your second toes. Reach your arms out to the sides and place your right hand on the barre for balance. Lift your heels off the floor and press evenly through the balls of your feet and base of each toe. Hold for 5 deep breaths.

MOVEMENT 1: Bend your knees, lowering your hips 1 inch as you keep your heels lifted.

MOVEMENT 2: Press into the balls of your feet and lift up 1 inch.

In this pose, letting your heels hover off the floor forces your legs, hips, and core to work hard at keeping you steady and stable. Play around by lifting your heels a little or a lot. You may find that one position helps you work even more deeply than the others.

RANGE: 1 inch
REPS: 30
TIME: 1 minute

GET DEEPER:

- Press evenly through the balls of your feet and the base of each toe.
- Draw your waist in as you lengthen all four sides of your torso.
- Engage the muscles in your arms.

MODIFICATIONS:

- To minimize foot or ankle discomfort, or for added balance, work with flat feet and focus on rooting all four corners of your feet.
- To minimize knee or hip discomfort, work higher or move your feet into a narrower stance.
- For an added balance challenge, try this without resting your hand on the barre.

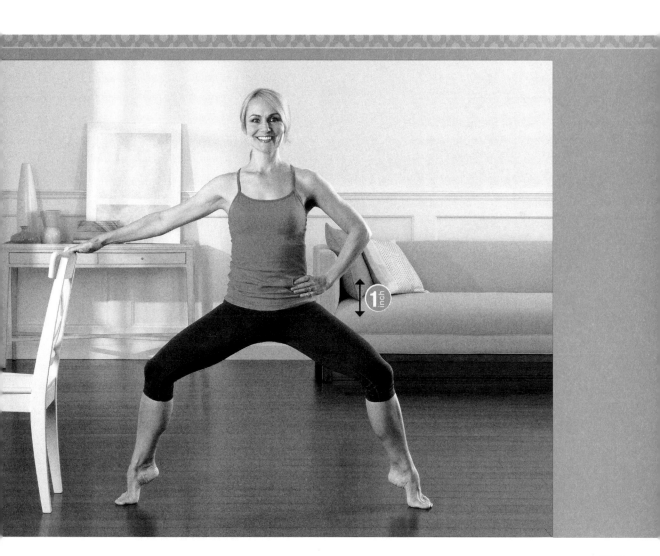

Starfish

SETUP: Stand in profile with your right hip next to your barre. Come to Horse Pose by stepping out wider than your hips with your feet turned out to 2 and 10 o'clock. Your shoulders are stacked over your hips and your core is engaged. Bend your knees and slide your back 6 inches down an imaginary wall. Your knees are over your ankles and in line with your second toes. Place your right hand on your barre and keep your left arm low. Hold for 5 deep breaths.

MOVEMENT 1: Press into your right foot and lift up and slightly over your barre. Lift and extend your left leg and sweep your left arm overhead.

MOVEMENT 2: Return to your setup position, lowering your lifted leg and arm and bending your knees 6 inches.

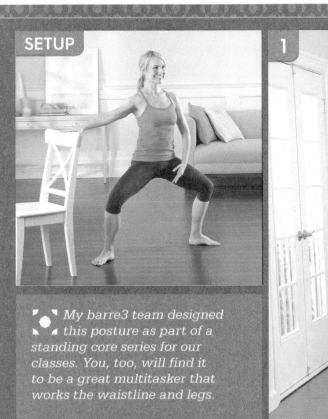

SETUP

1

◄●► My barre3 team designed this posture as part of a standing core series for our classes. You, too, will find it to be a great multitasker that works the waistline and legs.

GET DEEPER:

- Root through all four corners of your supporting foot.
- Draw your waist in and lengthen the side body.
- Reach strongly through your lifted arm.
- Engage your glutes as you lengthen your leg away from you and point your toes.

MODIFICATION:

- To minimize foot or ankle discomfort, or for extra balance, keep both feet rooted and extend your arm overhead as you lean to the side.

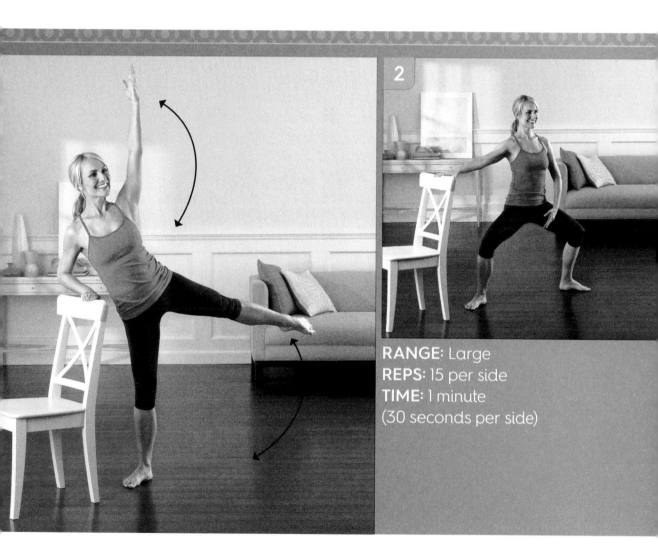

RANGE: Large
REPS: 15 per side
TIME: 1 minute
(30 seconds per side)

Carousel Horse

SETUP: Rest your hands lightly on the barre with your feet parallel and hip-width apart. Step your left foot back and bend both knees into a lunge and hold. Your right knee is directly over your right ankle. Your left knee is directly under your left hip. Keep your hips level and square, engage your core, and stack your shoulders directly over your hips. Hold for 5 deep breaths.

MOVEMENT 1: Lower your left knee 1 inch toward the floor. Your right knee stays directly over your ankle.

MOVEMENT 2: Press your feet into the floor and lift up 1 inch.

I named this posture Carousel Horse after watching my kids ride the carousel one day at the Oakland Zoo. As I do this exercise, I like to imagine a pole lifting me up to stay graceful and light.

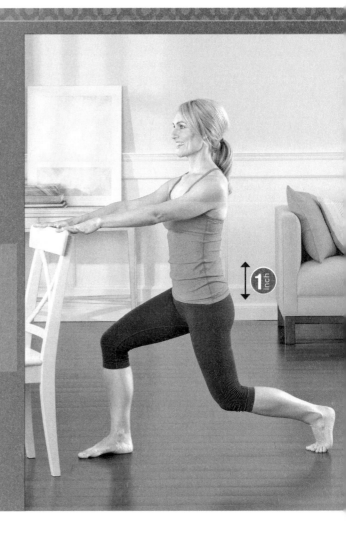

GET DEEPER:

- Root evenly through all four corners of your front foot and the base of each toe on your back foot.
- Draw your inner thighs inward toward your midline.
- Draw your waist in and lengthen your spine.
- Relax your shoulders down your back.

MODIFICATIONS:

- To minimize lower-back or knee discomfort, work higher with your back knee or place your back foot farther behind you.
- To minimize lower-back or knee discomfort, another option is to work with your upper body hinged slightly forward from the waistline (pictured below). This inclined position will take pressure off your back knee as you place more weight on your front foot.

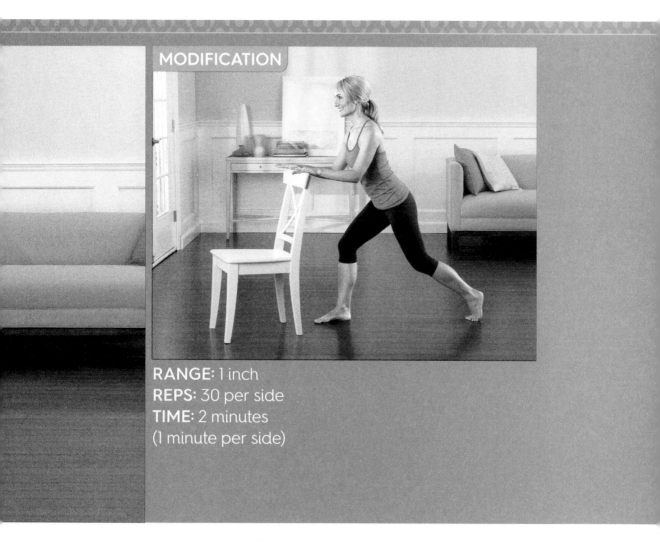

MODIFICATION

RANGE: 1 inch
REPS: 30 per side
TIME: 2 minutes
(1 minute per side)

Narrow Athletic V

SETUP: Bring your heels together and turn your legs out so your toes are 3 or 4 inches apart. Press your heels firmly together, then lift them slightly off the floor, coming onto the balls of your feet. Your hips stay level and square. Bend your knees over your second toes and lower your hips 6 inches. Your spine is long with your shoulders stacked over your hips. Rest your hand lightly on the barre (pictured below). Hold for 5 deep breaths.

MOVEMENT 1: Bend your knees to lower your hips 1 inch.

MOVEMENT 2: Press your heels together as you lift up 1 inch.

This pose works the tops of the legs, but it's also a sneaky way to work the seat: By pressing your heels firmly together, you also activate the glutes! The stance is much narrower than traditional ballet's first position. When you look down, you see the shape of a slice of pie in between your feet.

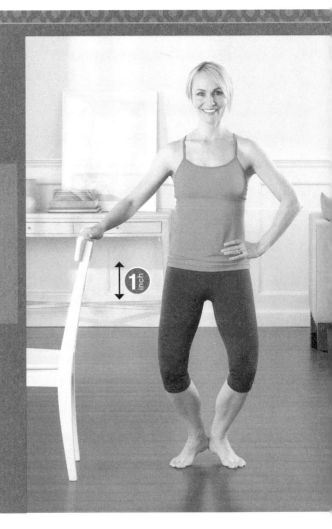

GET DEEPER:

- Press your heels more firmly together.
- Squeeze your inner thighs up and toward each other as you lift up 1 inch.
- Draw your waist in and focus on lengthening your spine.
- Relax your shoulders down your back.

MODIFICATIONS:

- To minimize foot or ankle discomfort, or for more stability, work with flat feet.
- To minimize knee or lower-back discomfort, work higher.
- Prop option: Place the core ball between your inner thighs and squeeze it as you lift up.
- Bring your palms together in prayer to challenge your balance (pictured below).

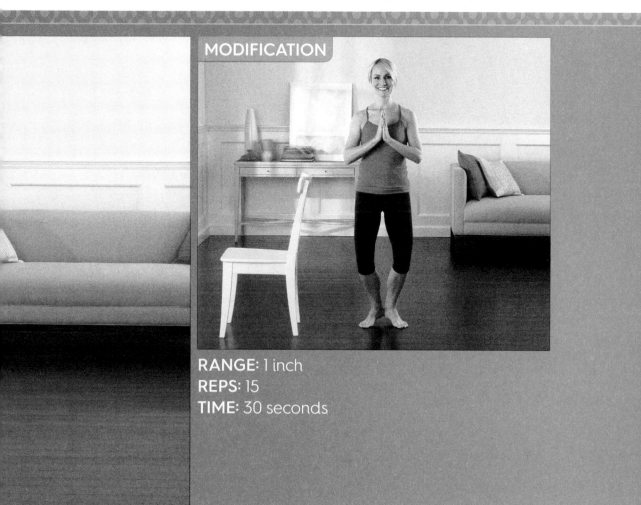

MODIFICATION

RANGE: 1 inch
REPS: 15
TIME: 30 seconds

Narrow Athletic V Twists

SETUP: Bring your heels together and turn your legs out so your toes are 3 or 4 inches apart. Press your heels firmly together, then lift them slightly off the floor, coming onto the balls of your feet. Your hips stay level and square. Bend your knees over your second toes and lower your hips 6 inches. Your spine is long with your shoulders stacked over your hips. Bend your elbows back by your sides with your hands on your hips. Hold for 5 deep breaths.

MOVEMENT 1: Keep your hips and legs still as you use your abs to twist your upper body to the right. At the same time extend your left arm forward and across your body.

MOVEMENT 2: Keep your core engaged and hips still as you twist your upper body to the left. At the same time, extend your right arm forward and across your body.

This posture is great for working your abdominals, especially your obliques, while you continue to work your seat and legs. The challenge is to keep your feet grounded and your hips still while twisting your upper body.

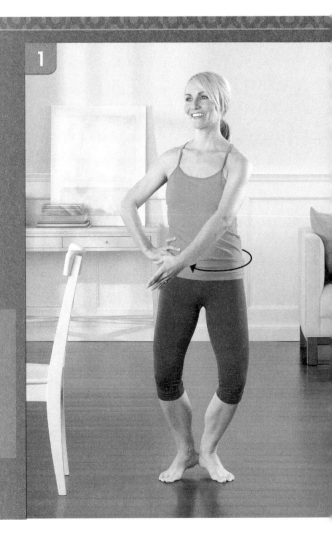

GET DEEPER:

- Press the balls of your feet firmly into the floor.
- Draw your waist in and engage your glutes to stabilize your pelvis.
- Firm your core in as you lengthen through the crown of your head.

MODIFICATIONS:

- To minimize foot or ankle discomfort, or for more stability, work with flat feet.
- To minimize knee or lower-back discomfort, work higher.
- For added balance, face the barre and alternate the hand resting on it.
- Prop option: For more inner-thigh work and hip stability, place the core ball between your inner thighs and gently squeeze it.

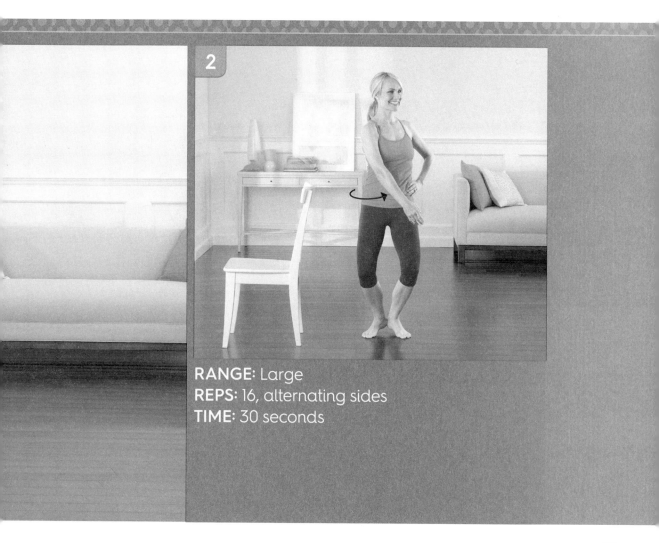

RANGE: Large
REPS: 16, alternating sides
TIME: 30 seconds

Sumo Squats

SETUP: Step your feet out slightly wider than your hips and turn your legs out so your toes point to 1 and 11 o'clock. Bend your knees and move your hips down and back into a squat. Your hands come together in front of your chest, and your knees are stacked over your ankles and in line with your second toes. Your spine is long, your abs are hugging in, and your shoulders are drawing down your back. Hold for 5 deep breaths.

MOVEMENT 1: Press into your feet and straighten your legs. At the same time, extend your arms overhead, palms facing in.

MOVEMENT 2: Bend your knees, reach your hips back, and bring your hands back in front of your chest, returning to your starting position.

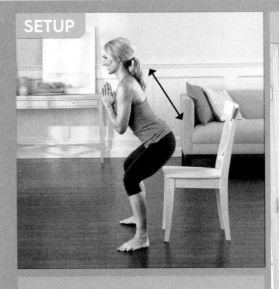

SETUP

1

This is one of my favorite exercises. It's found in most sports training and traditional gym settings, but it also fits into the barre3 way of training. By working deep in the glutes and legs, you strengthen the entire lower body.

GET DEEPER:

- Root all four corners of your feet evenly into the floor.
- Engage your seat muscles as you firm your inner thighs up and in.
- Draw your waist in.

MODIFICATIONS:

- To minimize knee or lower-back discomfort, work higher in Sumo.
- To minimize shoulder discomfort, keep your hands pressed together in front of your chest.
- Prop option: Use a chair to guide your form. Without actually sitting in it, sink your tailbone down toward the chair and hover your butt just above the seat, then return to standing.

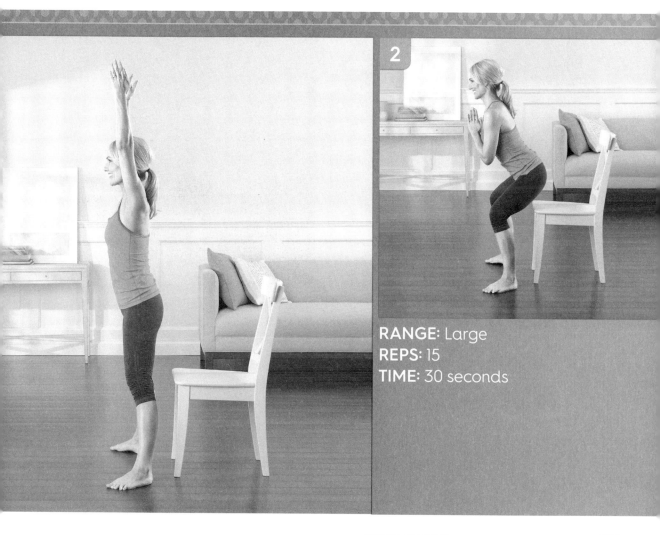

RANGE: Large
REPS: 15
TIME: 30 seconds

Power Leg

SETUP: Stand a forearm's distance from the barre. Place your feet hip-width apart with your toes, knees, and tops of your thighs pointed straight ahead. Place your palms lightly on the barre, lift your heels high, and root down into the balls of your feet. Bend your knees forward and slide your back down an imaginary wall. Keep your hips stacked over your ankles and your shoulders stacked over your hips, and engage your core muscles. Hold for 5 deep breaths.

MOVEMENT 1: Bend your knees, lowering your hips 1 inch as you keep your heels lifted.

MOVEMENT 2: Press into the balls of your feet and lift up 1 inch.

This posture tones and shapes the thighs while you work in an upright, neutral posture. It's sure to give you the famous barre3 earthquakes.

RANGE: 1 inch
REPS: 30
TIME: 1 minute

GET DEEPER:

- Press the base of each toe and the balls of your feet evenly into the floor.
- Engage your inner thighs.
- Firm in through your core to keep your torso upright.
- Relax your shoulders down your back.

MODIFICATIONS:

- To minimize knee or lower-back discomfort, work higher.
- To minimize knee or foot discomfort, lower your heels to a hover.
- Prop option: Place the core ball between your inner thighs to stabilize your knees and to add more inner-thigh and core work.

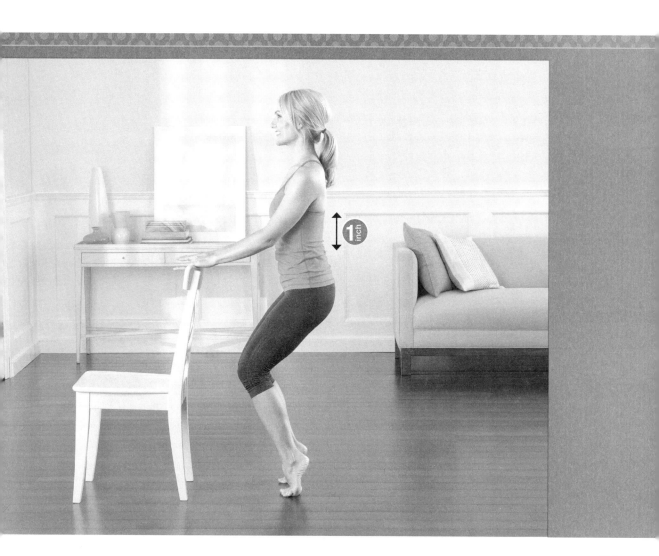

Standing Leg Lift

SETUP: Stand with your hands resting lightly on the barre and your feet hip-width apart. Extend your left leg back, pointing your foot and lifting your toes a few inches off the floor. Keep your standing knee soft, your hips square, your abs drawn in, and your lower back long. Relax your shoulders down your back. Hold for 5 deep breaths.

MOVEMENT 1: Engage your left hamstring and glutes and lift your left leg up 1 inch.

MOVEMENT 2: Lower your left leg 1 inch.

This posture is inspired by traditional ballet exercises used to strengthen the glutes. We do this by working in small, controlled movements and by keeping the abs tight and the lower back long.

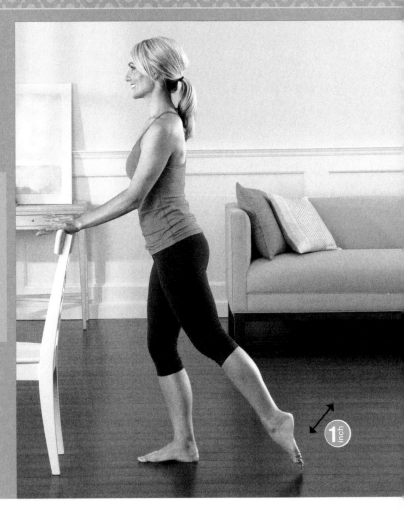

GET DEEPER:

- Draw your standing inner thigh up and in to stay upright and lifted out of your standing hip.
- Engage your core to keep your hips still and level.
- Spiral your extended leg inward so your knee points toward the floor.
- Engage your glutes of your extended leg as you lengthen your leg back behind you and point your toes.

MODIFICATION:

- To minimize lower-back discomfort, lean the upper body forward in an inclined position (pictured below).

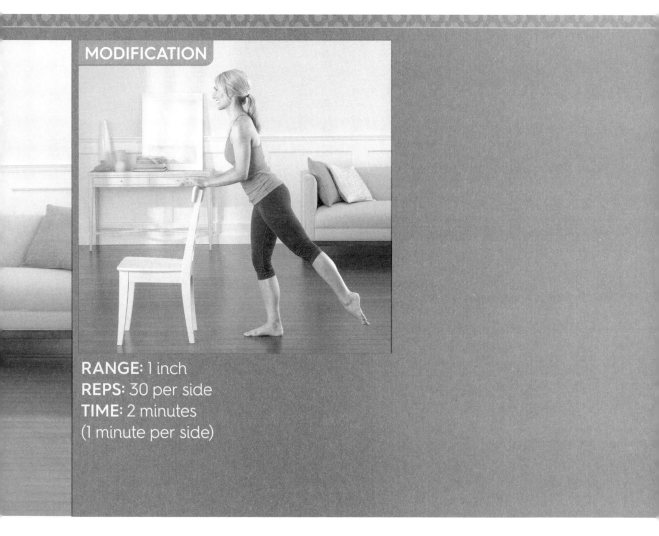

MODIFICATION

RANGE: 1 inch
REPS: 30 per side
TIME: 2 minutes
(1 minute per side)

Plank

Place your palms shoulder-width apart on the barre. Step your feet back and tilt forward with your heels, hips, and shoulders in one long line, keeping a neutral spine. Your body will be in a traditional plank position but with your hands on the barre, not the floor. Hold for 1 minute.

Do these on a sturdy surface like a wall-mounted counter or kitchen island.

Plank is one of the best exercises to strengthen the muscles of the core. We modify Plank by doing it at the barre. This allows us to develop long, lean muscles without putting additional pressure on the wrists, shoulders, and lower back.

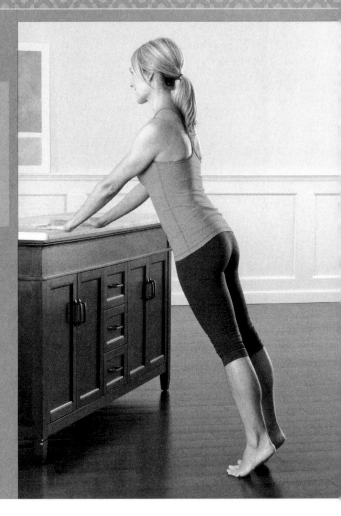

GET DEEPER:

- Press the base of each finger and the base of your thumbs into the barre.
- Widen your shoulders down your back.
- Engage your core, keeping your hips level.
- Reach up through the crown of your head and down through your tailbone and heels.

MODIFICATIONS:

- To minimize shoulder, neck, or wrist discomfort, step closer to the barre.
- For greater resistance, take Plank to the floor. Place your hands directly under your shoulders. Extend your legs behind you with the balls of your feet rooted to the floor (pictured below).
- Prop option: Place the core ball between your inner thighs and firm up and in to connect deeper with your inner thighs and your core.

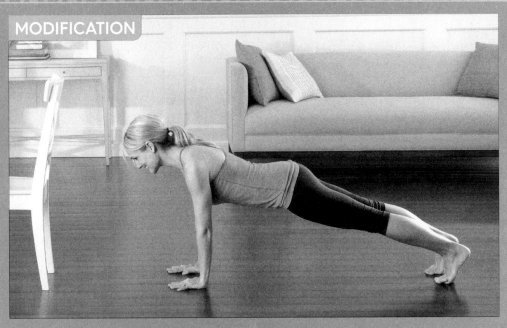

MODIFICATION

RANGE: Hold
REPS: 1
TIME: 1 minute

Triceps Foldover

Place your elbows on the barre and press your palms together. Walk your feet back and underneath your hips. Draw your head down and rest your forehead on the barre between your elbows. Engage your core and lengthen your spine. Let your chest fall slightly between your shoulders as you open your shoulders and chest. Hold for 5 deep breaths.

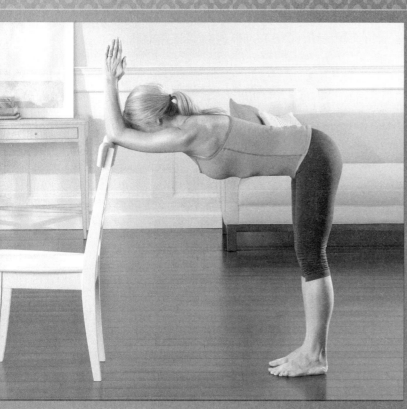

Do this on a sturdy surface like a wall-mounted counter or kitchen island for additional support.

This stretch opens up the shoulders, chest, hamstrings, and calves.

MODIFICATION:
• Bring your palms back to your shoulders for a deeper triceps stretch.

RANGE: Hold
REPS: 1
TIME: 1 minute

IT Band Stretch with a Twist

Place your palms shoulder-width apart on your barre. Step back into a Foldover position (1). Your feet are directly below your hips and your arms stretched out in front of you with palms resting on the barre. Engage your core and lengthen your spine. Relax your shoulders down your back. Bend your right knee and lean into your left hip (2). Draw your right shoulder toward the floor as you twist by reaching your right palm toward your left ankle (3). Hold for 5 deep breaths, then switch sides.

This stretch lengthens the side of the hip and leg by stretching the IT band, which runs along the outside of the thigh. The twist releases the spine while opening the chest and back. Your hamstrings and calves also release in this gentle forward fold.

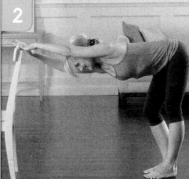

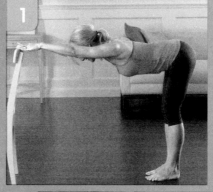

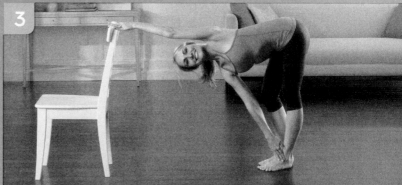

MODIFICATION:

- **To minimize lower-back discomfort, keep both hands on the barre during the twist.**

RANGE: Hold
REPS: 1 per side
TIME: 1 minute (30 seconds per side)

Crescent Lunge with Chest Opener

Step your hips up to the barre with your feet hip-width apart and your hands resting on the barre. Step your left foot back, extending your left leg in a lunge. Bend your right knee directly over your ankle. Hold your weight evenly through both feet and firm in through your inner thighs. Level and square your hips and engage your core. Sweep your arms back behind you like a cape, interlace your fingers, and squeeze your shoulder blades together as you lift your chest. Optionally, gaze up the wall in front of you, gently arching your upper back. Hold for 5 deep breaths, then switch sides.

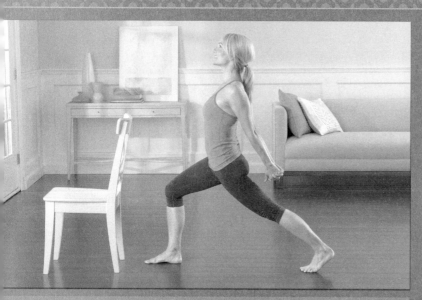

This stretch opens the fronts of the thighs, the hip flexors, and the chest. It's a great way to combat the slumped-over position so many of us assume when sitting.

GET DEEPER:

- Draw your tailbone down toward the floor while you pull your lower belly in.
- Relax your shoulders down your back.
- Draw your inner thighs in toward your midline.

MODIFICATIONS:

- For extra stability, keep your palms on the barre.
- To minimize neck, shoulder, or back discomfort, keep your arms reaching back like a cape and keep your gaze forward.
- To minimize lower-back or hip discomfort, scoot your back foot in and work higher.

RANGE: Hold
REPS: 1 per side
TIME: 1 minute (30 seconds per side)

Heel to Seat Stretch

With your right hand on the barre, stand tall, bending your left knee back and holding on to your left ankle with your left hand. Gently pull your heel in toward your seat. Soften your right knee, draw your inner thighs toward each other, and draw your abs in. Hold for 5 deep breaths, then switch sides.

GET DEEPER:

- **Root evenly through all four corners of your standing foot.**
- **Engage your core and lengthen your tailbone down to keep your hips level.**
- **Draw your bent knee gently behind your standing leg to deepen the stretch.**

This stretch lengthens the fronts of the thighs, the quadriceps muscles. It also reinforces an upright posture by opening up the shoulders and the hip flexors.

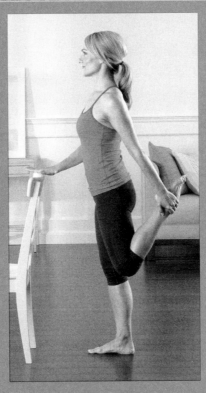

RANGE: Hold
REPS: 1 per side
TIME: 1 minute
(30 seconds per side)

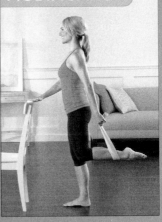

MODIFICATION

MODIFICATIONS:

- **If holding on to your ankle isn't an option for you, then grab your pant leg or use a yoga strap (or a belt): Loop the strap around your shin and hold both ends behind you as you would your ankle (pictured above).**
- **Lift your opposite hand into the air for a balance challenge.**

Figure 4

Step an arm's distance from the barre. Cross your left ankle over your right knee and press your hips back as if you were sitting in a chair. Place your hands lightly on the barre. Flex your left foot. Make sure your right knee is directly over your right ankle, your hips are level, belly is engaged, spine is long, and shoulders are down your back. Hold for 5 deep breaths, then switch sides.

GET DEEPER:

• Firm your belly in as you melt your shoulders down your back.

• Hips stay level as you reach your seat back and draw your bent knee down.

This is one of my favorite stretches to open up the hips, glutes, and back.

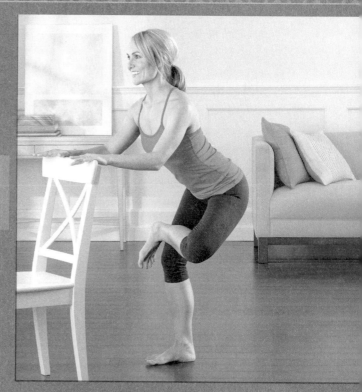

RANGE: Hold
REPS: 1 per side
TIME: 1 MINUTE
(30 seconds per side)

Raising the Barre

ERIN DINEEN

AGE: 31 POUNDS LOST: 15 INCHES LOST: 11¼ *including 2¾ from her waist*

I have been overweight most of my life. In 2006, my mom and I signed up to do Weight Watchers together. Over the next 2 years, I lost about 45 pounds. I also began running, and I got hooked. In 2009, I ran a few big races including a full marathon. I was super-active, but because I was eating whatever I wanted—and because that year was a hard on me in terms of work and relationships—I gained back most of the weight I had lost.

Over the next few years, I made some changes to my personal life that helped me feel healthier on the inside. I continued to work out, doing Zumba, indoor cycling, and running. I also went on a few different diets. They were all successful while they lasted (anywhere from 2 weeks to a month), but I always gave up.

I was excited to be picked for the Love Your Lower Body test panel. I noticed big changes in how I thought about my day from the get-go. I realized that when I planned my meals ahead of time, shopping for groceries and adding leftovers to my eating routine, I didn't have to

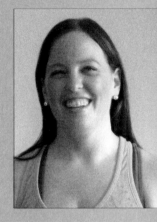

spend a lot of time thinking about food and could focus on everything else in my life. I also learned how this plan is a lifestyle as opposed to a diet. I can still treat myself or splurge, but for the most part, I know what my body wants and needs. I have learned to incorporate healthy eating habits into my life instead of changing how I live in order to follow a diet.

Because of the addition of these 10-minute workouts to my training routine, I am in better running shape—even though I'm actually running less! Barre3 gives me the balance of core strength, weight training, and endurance that I need to succeed in many aspects of my life. I have less lower-back pain currently because my posture has improved as a result of my core being stronger. I stand taller, and I feel like I've really gained my confidence back. I just ran another race, and I was blown away by my time.

These days I'm happy, healthy, and full of energy. I wake up early in the morning to work out and I really enjoy it. I still have a ways to go, but I know I can keep this going. As I make choices about my future, I am doing so with a clearer focus and greater feelings of peace because of the balance this program has brought to my life. I have gained physical and mental strength over the past few months, and I have the Love Your Lower Body program to thank for that.

I LOVE MY LOWER BODY *because:*

Stairs are *not* a problem. My jeans look great! I can run farther. My lower body gets me through long workouts without any pain.

Chapter 6

7

More Weeks to LOVE Your LOWER BODY

AFTER YOUR FIRST WEEK ON THE PLAN, YOU'VE SEEN HOW SIMPLE and effective the 10 Tranformative Minutes can be. While you can get great results over 8 weeks just doing this workout, there are plenty of reasons to shake it up.

New exercises and sequences will continue to challenge your muscles in new and different ways. Think back to the start of Week 1. The first day you did the 10 Transformative Minutes routine, you probably found it quite challenging. But by the end of the week, you likely felt you were getting the hang of it. Building muscle and becoming more proficient at these exercises is great—but it's important to keep challenging your muscles. Otherwise, the routines may become a little less effective as your body learns to anticipate the movement. Not only will your muscles benefit from new routines, but so will your brain! New challenges help you stay interested and focused as you gain strength, endurance, and flexibility.

I have designed the next 7 weeks to gradually work your different muscle groups, adding your arms and upper-back muscles at times, challenging your core at others, and really targeting your glutes, too.

In this chapter, I will take you through the remaining 7 weeks of the plan. Each week adds a new element to your Love Your Lower Body routine. Let's get started!

Week 2

Full-Body Blast

Welcome to Week 2. By now, you should be fully on board with the 10 Transformative Minutes. You'll continue to focus on this routine, but I offer new options to help you dial up the intensity. To the basic 10 Transformative Minutes, I add movements designed to target your upper body and core, creating a brand-new 10-minute routine I call the Full-Body Blast.

In addition to using a sturdy barre (such as your countertop), you have the option to use light handheld weights. Most of my clients start with 1-pound weights and then work toward 2-pounders. If you don't have weights, you can still get a good workout: The movement is designed to tone your upper body by using your own body weight as resistance.

This week you also add an extra workout 4 days a week, so that some days you'll fit in 40 minutes of exercise. I invite you to break up your 40 minutes, doing one round of the 10 Transformative Minutes by itself, then grouping the other 30 minutes of exercise into a seamless progression from the 10 Transformative Minutes to the Standing Stretch to the Full-Body Blast and back to the Standing Stretch. The stretch segments between the two workouts give you an extra chance to catch your breath, recover, and prepare for more movement.

Ready for Week 2? Review this workout summary and then dive into the following pages to learn the Full-Body Blast.

Week 2

DAY 1	DAY 2	DAY 3	DAY 4	DAY 5	DAY 6	DAY 7
10 min	40 min	40 min	10 min	40 min	Rest	40 min

On Days 1 and 4, you will do the 10 Transformative Minutes.

On Days 2, 3, 5, and 7, you will do the 10 Transformative Minutes with the Standing Stretch, new Full-Body Blast, and Standing Stretch again.

Days 2, 3, 5 & 7

10 Transformative Minutes

Horse Pose Pliés p.100

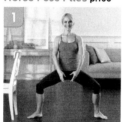

Horse Pose with Heels Lifted p.102

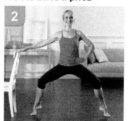

Starfish p.104

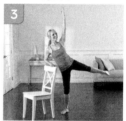

Carousel Horse p.106

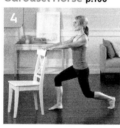

Narrow Athletic V p.108

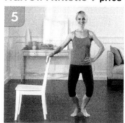

Narrow Athletic V Twists p.110

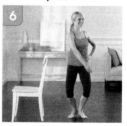

Sumo Squats p.112

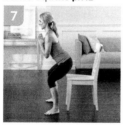

Power Leg p.114

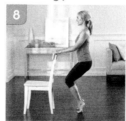

Standing Leg Lift p.116

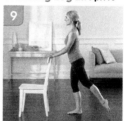

Plank p.118

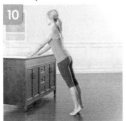

Standing Stretch

Triceps Foldover p.120

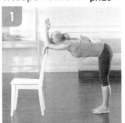

IT Band Stretch with a Twist p.121

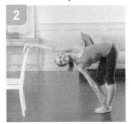

Crescent Lunge with Chest Opener p.122

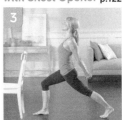

Heel to Seat Stretch p.123

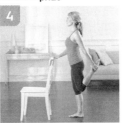

Figure 4 p.124

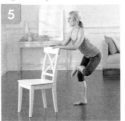

Full-Body Blast

New!

Horse Pose Pliés with Snow Angels p.134

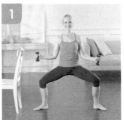

Horse Pose with Elbow Nudges p.136

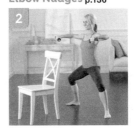

Starfish with Lat/Oblique Pulls p.138

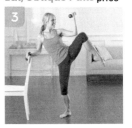

(continued)

Days 2, 3, 5 & 7 *(cont'd)*

Full-Body Blast (cont'd)

Incline Carousel Horse with Biceps Curls p.140

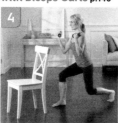

Incline Carousel Horse with Triceps Presses p.142

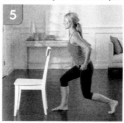

Narrow Athletic V with Rhomboid Squeezes p.144

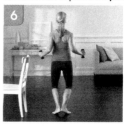

Narrow Athletic V Twists with Weights p.146

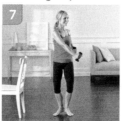

Sumo Squats with Wide Rows p.148

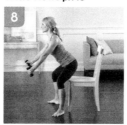

Power Leg with Abdominal Scoops p.150

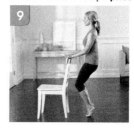

Standing Leg Lifts with Mini Triceps Pushups p.152

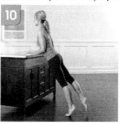

Wide Pushups p.154

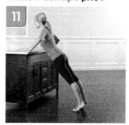

Triceps Foldover p.120

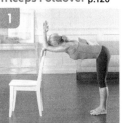

IT Band Stretch with a Twist p.121

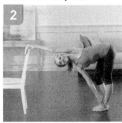

Crescent Lunge with Chest Opener p.122

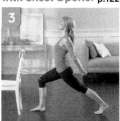

Heel to Seat Stretch p.123

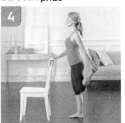

Figure 4 p.124

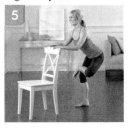

Horse Pose Pliés
with Snow Angels

SETUP: Hold a weight in each hand. Come to Horse Pose by stepping out wider than your hips with your feet turned out to 2 and 10 o'clock. Your shoulders are stacked over your hips and your core is engaged. Bend your knees and slide your back 6 inches down an imaginary wall. Your knees are over your ankles and in line with your second toes. Your elbows are at your waist with your palms facing forward. Hold for 5 deep breaths.

MOVEMENT 1: Push down with your feet and straighten your legs. At the same time, circle your arms to the sides and overhead.

MOVEMENT 2: Bend your knees and lower your hips to the starting position as you bring your elbows back to your waist.

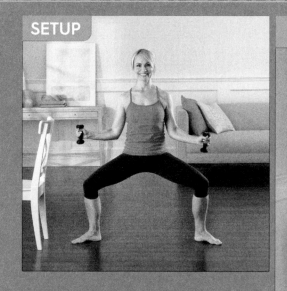

GET DEEPER:

- Relax your shoulders down your back.
- Feel resistance as you move your arms.
- Engage your core, draw your inner thighs up and in, and engage your glutes.
- Root evenly through all four corners of your feet into the floor and imagine you're pulling your heels toward each other.

MODIFICATION:

- To minimize neck or shoulder discomfort, lower your arms to shoulder-level height.

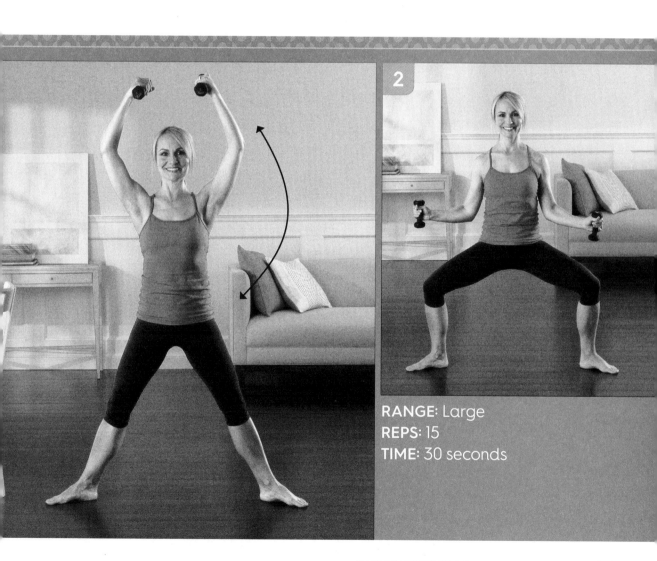

RANGE: Large
REPS: 15
TIME: 30 seconds

Horse Pose with Elbow Nudges

SETUP: Hold a weight in each hand. Come to Horse Pose by stepping out wider than your hips with your feet turned out to 2 and 10 o'clock. Your shoulders are stacked over your hips and your core is engaged. Slide your back 6 inches down an imaginary wall, bending your knees over your ankles so they're in line with your second toes. Lift your arms to your sides, then bend your elbows, pointing your forearms forward. Hold for 5 deep breaths.

MOVEMENT 1: Lower your hips 1 inch, keeping your core engaged. At the same time, press your elbows back 1 inch by engaging the muscles in your upper back.

MOVEMENT 2: Press into your feet to lift up 1 inch, bringing your arms 1 inch forward.

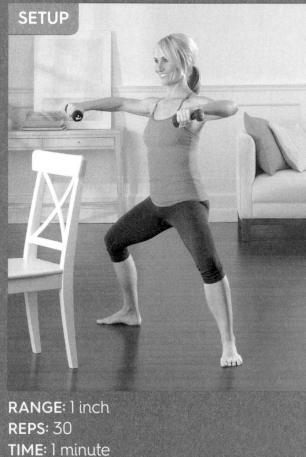

SETUP

RANGE: 1 inch
REPS: 30
TIME: 1 minute

GET DEEPER:

- Press evenly through your feet.
- Firm your inner thighs up and in and engage your glutes, finding a sense of lift.
- Relax your shoulders down your back to keep a long neck and spine.

MODIFICATION:

- To minimize neck or shoulder discomfort, lower your elbows slightly.

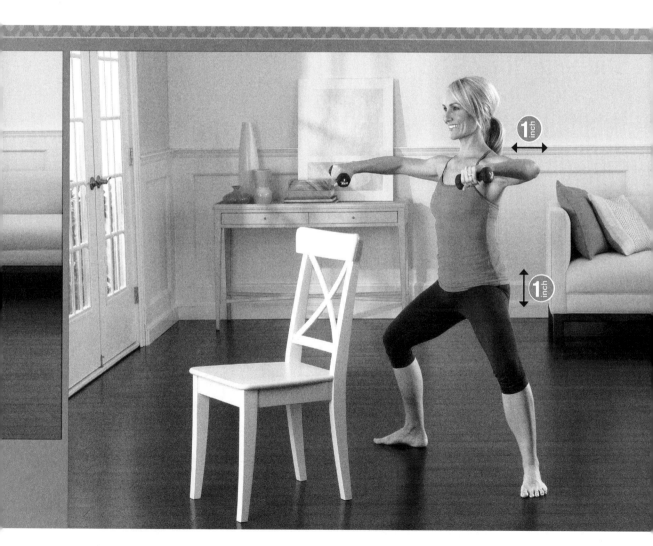

Starfish with Lat/Oblique Pull

SETUP: Stand in profile with your right hip next to the barre. Come to Horse Pose by stepping out wider than your hips with your feet turned out to 2 and 10 o'clock. Your shoulders are stacked over your hips and your core is engaged. Bend your knees and slide your back 6 inches down an imaginary wall. Your knees are over your ankles and in line with your second toes. Place your right hand on the barre; hold a weight in your left hand and keep it low. Hold for 5 deep breaths.

MOVEMENT 1: Press into your right foot and lift up and slightly over the barre. Lift and extend your left leg and sweep your left arm overhead.

MOVEMENT 2: Pull your left elbow and left knee toward each other while firming your core.

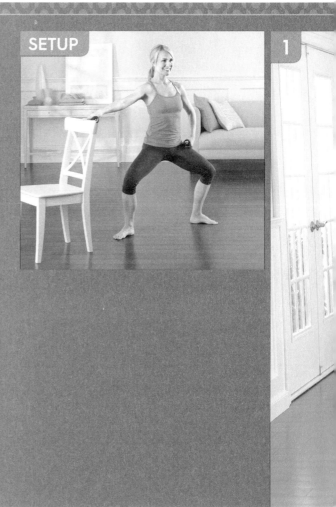

GET DEEPER:

- Root through all four corners of your supporting foot and point the lifted toes.
- Draw your waist in and lengthen the side body.
- Reach strongly through your top arm and keep your shoulder down your back.
- Engage your glutes as you lengthen your leg away.
- Find resistance as you pull your knee and elbow in and cinch in through the waistline.

MODIFICATIONS:

- To dial down the intensity, work your upper body only, keeping both feet on the floor.
- To minimize neck or shoulder discomfort, keep your working arm at shoulder height.

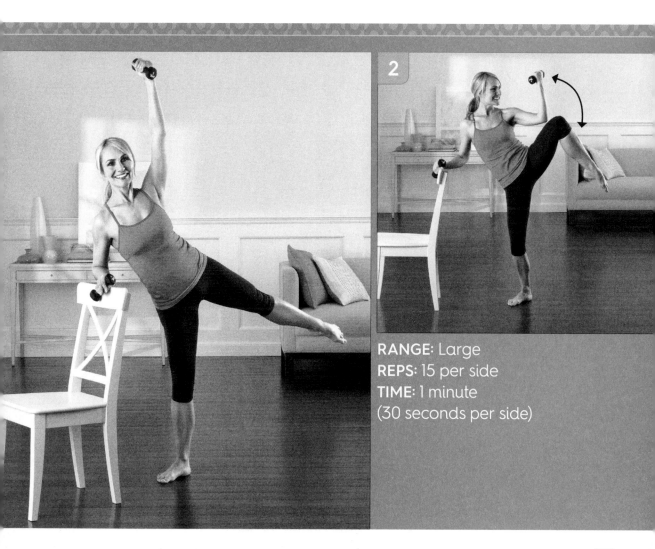

RANGE: Large
REPS: 15 per side
TIME: 1 minute
(30 seconds per side)

Incline Carousel Horse
with Biceps Curls

SETUP: Hold a weight in each hand. Step your left foot back and bend both knees into a lunge and hold. Your right knee is directly over your right ankle. Your left knee is directly under your left hip. Keep your hips level and square, engage your core, and hinge your torso slightly forward, pressing into your right foot and taking some of the weight off the ball of your left foot. Reach your arms out in front of you in a low V, palms facing up, and relax your shoulders down your back. Hold for 5 deep breaths.

MOVEMENT 1: Lower your left knee 1 inch toward the floor. Your right knee stays directly over your ankle. At the same time, pull your palms toward your shoulders, keeping your elbows still.

MOVEMENT 2: Press your feet into the floor to lift up 1 inch as you extend your arms to the starting position.

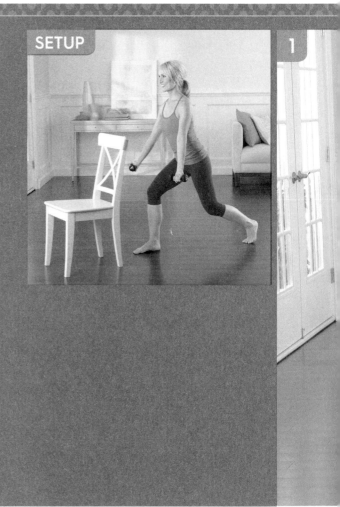

GET DEEPER:

- Root evenly through all four corners of your front foot and the base of each toe on your back foot.
- Firm your inner thighs in toward your midline.
- Draw your abdominals in and lengthen your spine.
- Relax your shoulders down your back.
- Feel resistance as you move your arms.

MODIFICATIONS:

- To minimize neck or shoulder discomfort, work with your arms closer to your body.
- To minimize knee discomfort, stand in primary posture and focus on the biceps curls.

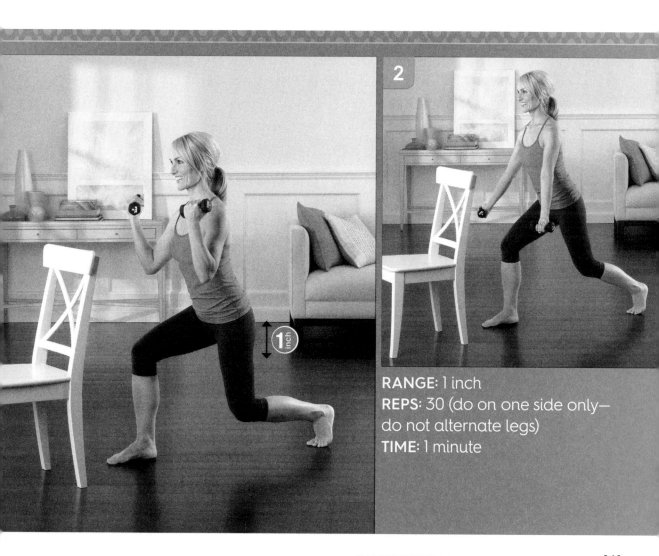

RANGE: 1 inch
REPS: 30 (do on one side only—do not alternate legs)
TIME: 1 minute

Incline Carousel Horse with Triceps Presses

SETUP: Hold a weight in each hand. Step your right foot back and bend both knees into a lunge. (You are stepping back with the leg opposite the one used in Incline Carousel Horse with Biceps Curls.) Your left knee is directly over your left ankle. Your right knee is directly under your right hip. Keep your hips level and square, engage your core, and hinge your torso slightly forward, pressing into your front foot and taking some of the weight off your back foot. Reach your arms behind you like a cape, palms turned toward your hips. Relax your shoulders down your back. Hold for 5 deep breaths.

MOVEMENT 1: Lower your back knee 1 inch toward the floor. Your front knee stays directly over your ankle. At the same time, gently bend your elbows.

MOVEMENT 2: Press your feet into the floor to lift up 1 inch as you extend your arms to the starting position.

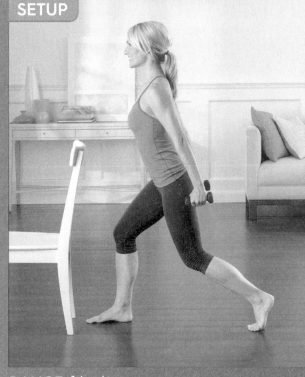

SETUP

RANGE: 1 inch
REPS: 30 (do on one side only—do not alternate legs)
TIME: 1 minute

GET DEEPER:

- Root evenly through all four corners of your front foot and the base of each toe on your back foot.
- Draw your inner thighs toward your midline.
- Draw your waist in and lengthen your spine.
- Relax your shoulders down your back.
- Find resistance as you strongly reach long with your arms.

MODIFICATIONS:

- To minimize neck or shoulder discomfort, lower your arms.
- To minimize knee discomfort, eliminate the knee bend.

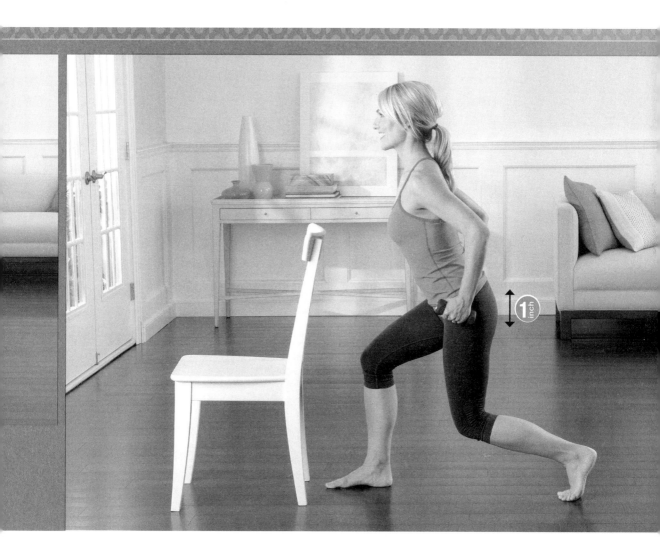

Narrow Athletic V with Rhomboid Squeezes

SETUP: Hold a weight in each hand. Bring your heels together and turn your legs out so your toes are 3 or 4 inches apart. Press your heels firmly together and lift them slightly off the floor, coming onto the balls of your feet. Your hips stay level and square. Bend your knees over your second toes and lower your hips 6 inches. Your spine is long with your shoulders stacked over your hips. Bend your elbows in next to your waist and turn your palms forward. Hold for 5 deep breaths.

MOVEMENT 1: Bend your knees and lower your hips 1 inch. At the same time, squeeze your shoulder blades together and draw your elbows behind you 1 inch.

MOVEMENT 2: Lift up 1 inch, opening your arms to the starting position.

RANGE: 1 inch
REPS: 15
TIME: 30 seconds

GET DEEPER:

- Press your heels firmly together.
- Engage your inner thighs up and toward each other as you lift up 1 inch.
- Draw your waist in and focus on lengthening your spine.
- Keep your ribs down as you firm your shoulder blades together.

MODIFICATIONS:

- To minimize discomfort in your feet or ankles, work with flat feet for more stability.
- To minimize discomfort in your lower back or knees, work higher and with less bend in your knees.
- Prop option: Place the core ball between your inner thighs to stabilize your knees and to add more inner-thigh and core work.

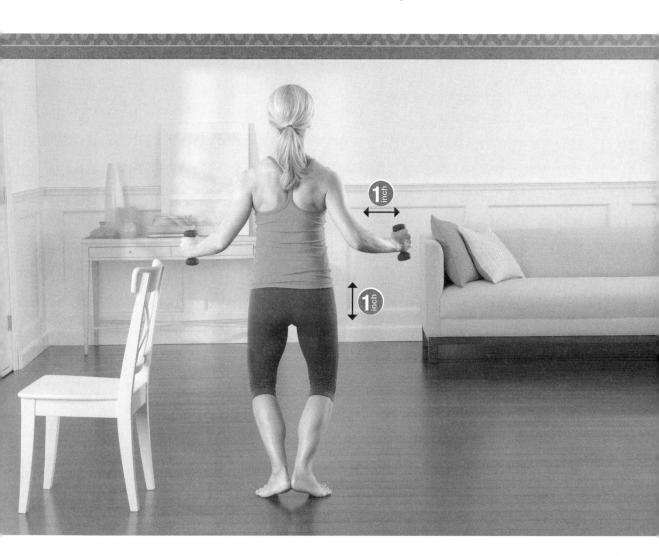

Narrow Athletic V Twists with Weights

SETUP: Hold a weight in each hand. Bring your heels together and turn your legs out so your toes are 3 or 4 inches apart. Press your heels firmly together. (Optional: Lift them slightly off the floor, coming onto the balls of your feet.) Your hips stay level and square. Bend your knees over your second toes and lower your hips 6 inches. Your spine is long with your shoulders stacked over your hips. Relax your shoulders down your back. Bend your elbows back by your sides. Hold for 5 deep breaths.

MOVEMENT 1: Keep your hips and legs still as you use your abs to twist your upper body to the right. At the same time, extend your left arm forward and across your body.

MOVEMENT 2: Keep your core engaged and hips still as you twist your upper body to the left. At the same time, extend your right arm forward and across your body.

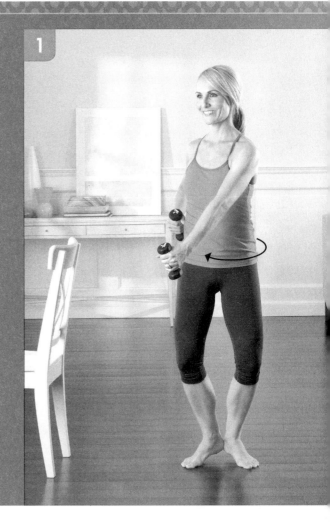

GET DEEPER:

- Press the balls of your feet firmly into the floor and squeeze your heels.
- Draw your waist in and engage your glutes to stabilize your pelvis.
- Lengthen through your reaching arm and pull back through the opposite elbow.
- Find resistance as you move your arms and twist from your core.

MODIFICATIONS:

- To minimize discomfort in your feet or ankles, work with flat feet for more stability.
- To minimize discomfort in your lower back or knees, work higher and with less bend in your knees.
- Prop option: For more inner-thigh work and hip stability, place the core ball between your inner thighs and gently squeeze it.

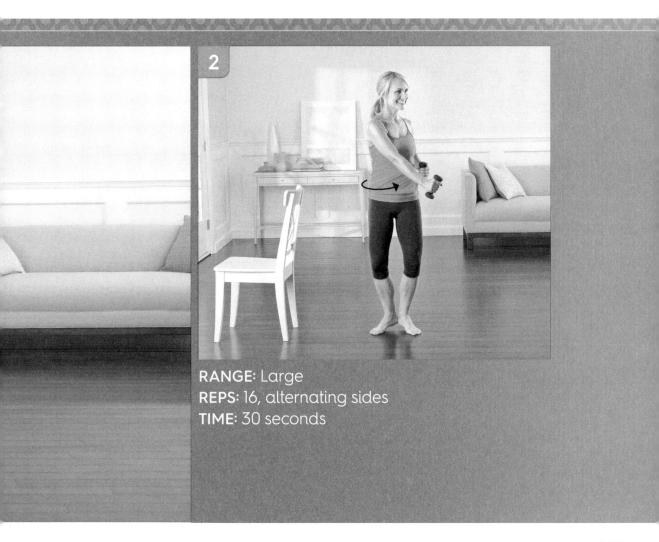

RANGE: Large
REPS: 16, alternating sides
TIME: 30 seconds

Sumo Squats with Wide Rows

SETUP: Hold a weight in each hand. Step your feet out slightly wider than your hips and turn your legs out so your toes point to 1 and 11 o'clock. Bend your knees and move your hips down and back into a squat. Your spine is long, your abs are hugging in, and your shoulders are drawing down your back. Reach your arms forward to form a low V, palms facing each other. Hold for 5 deep breaths.

MOVEMENT 1: Press into your feet and straighten your legs. At the same time, bend your elbows back by your waist and squeeze your shoulder blades together.

MOVEMENT 2: Bend your knees, reach your hips back, and reach your hands forward into a low V, returning to the setup position.

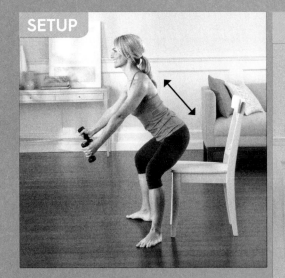

SETUP

1

GET DEEPER:

- Root all four corners of your feet evenly to the floor.
- Engage your glutes and draw your inner thighs up and in.
- Draw your waist in.
- Relax your shoulders down your back.
- Feel the resistance as you press your arms and and firm your elbows in.

MODIFICATIONS:

- To minimize knee or lower-back discomfort, work higher or smaller.
- Prop option: Use a chair to guide your form. Without actually sitting in it, sink your tailbone down toward the seat, hovering just above it, and then return to standing.

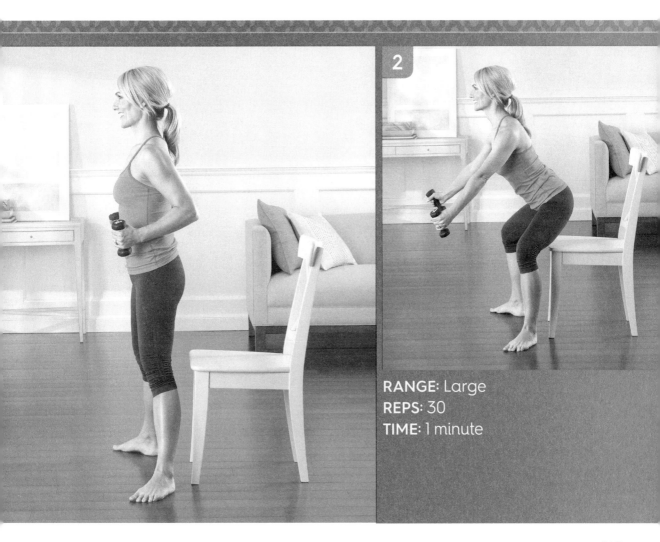

RANGE: Large
REPS: 30
TIME: 1 minute

Power Leg with Abdominal Scoops

SETUP: Stand a forearm's distance from the barre. Place your feet hip-width apart with your toes, knees, and tops of your thighs pointed straight ahead. Place your palms lightly on the barre, lift your heels high, and root down into the balls of your feet. Bend your knees forward and slide your back down an imaginary wall. Keep your hips stacked over your ankles, your shoulders stacked over your hips, and your core firm. Hold for 5 deep breaths.

MOVEMENT 1: Scoop your lower belly, rounding your lower back and tilting your pelvis up.

MOVEMENT 2: Keeping your core engaged, return your hips to neutral alignment.

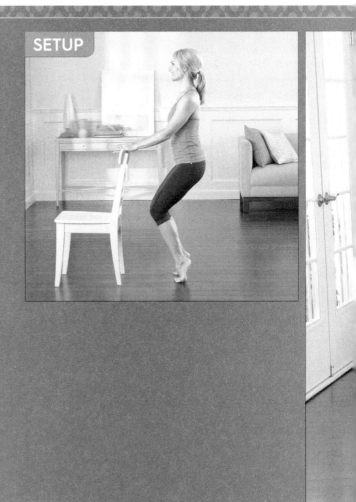

SETUP

GET DEEPER:

- Press the balls of your feet and the base of each toe evenly into the floor.
- Engage your inner thighs.
- Firm in through your core to keep your torso upright.
- Widen your shoulders down your back.

MODIFICATIONS:

- To minimize knee, foot, or lower-back discomfort, work with flat feet. Scoop through your lower belly and repeat.
- Prop option: Place the core ball between your inner thighs to stabilize your knees and to add more inner-thigh and core work.

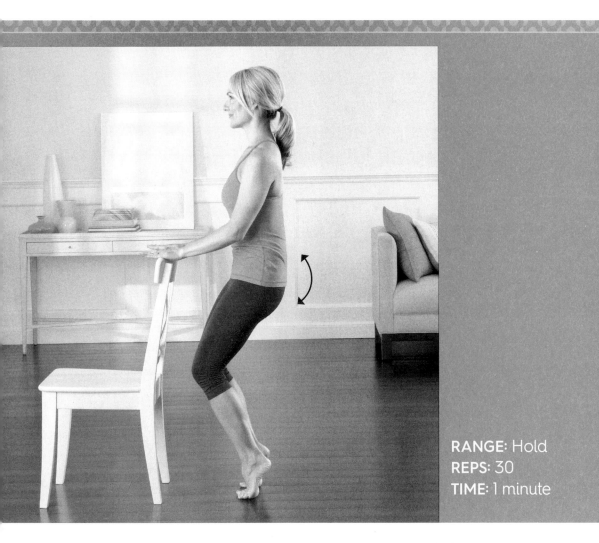

RANGE: Hold
REPS: 30
TIME: 1 minute

Standing Leg Lifts
with Mini Triceps Pushups

SETUP: Place your palms shoulder-width apart on the barre. Stand a full arm's distance from the barre. Lift your heels 1 inch and find a Plank position. Your shoulders, hips, and heels are in line. Press your palms down, relax your shoulders, and draw your core in. Extend your right leg back, pointing your foot and lifting your toes a few inches off the floor. Keep your left knee soft, your hips square, and your lower back long. Hold for 5 deep breaths.

Do these on a sturdy surface like a wall-mounted counter or kitchen island.

MOVEMENT 1: Bend your elbows halfway, squeezing them against your waist and lowering your body in Plank position.

MOVEMENT 2: Extend your arms, coming back to the starting position. Your right leg stays extended behind you.

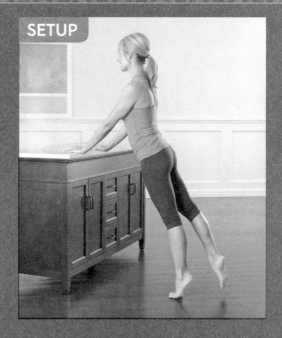

SETUP

GET DEEPER:

- Root the ball of your standing foot evenly to the floor.
- Draw your standing inner thigh in and up to stay upright and out of your standing hip.
- Spiral the inner thigh of your extended leg inward and draw in your waist.
- Firm in through your glutes as you strongly reach your leg behind you with a pointed toe.
- Press your palms firmly into the barre to engage the backs of your arms.
- Melt your shoulders down your back.

MODIFICATIONS:

- To minimize lower-back discomfort, hinge forward slightly and work in an inclined position.
- To minimize foot or ankle discomfort, work with a flat foot.
- To minimize neck or shoulder discomfort, work higher in the pushup or step closer to the barre.

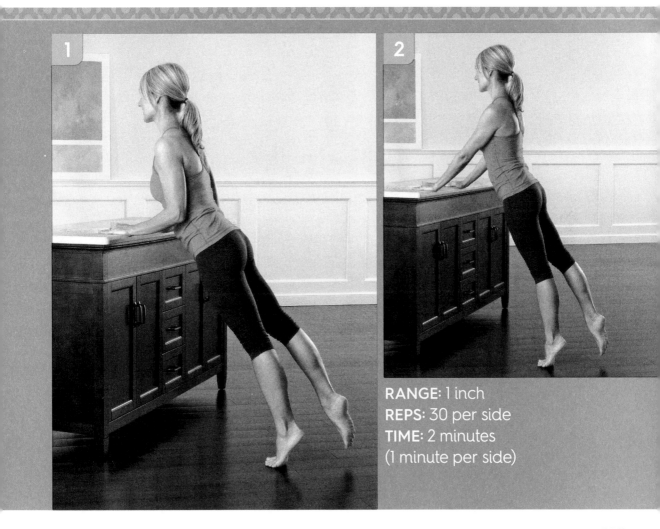

RANGE: 1 inch
REPS: 30 per side
TIME: 2 minutes
(1 minute per side)

Wide Pushups

SETUP: Place your palms about 2 feet apart on the barre. Step your feet back until your heels, hips, and shoulders are in one long line and you have a neutral spine. Your body will be in a traditional Plank position but with your hands on the barre, not the floor. Press your palms down, relax your shoulders down your back, draw your core in, and reach your heels down. Hold for 5 deep breaths.

Do these on a sturdy surface like a wall-mounted counter or kitchen island.

MOVEMENT 1: Bend your elbows halfway, lowering them so they're in line with your wrists. Your body is still in a Plank position.

MOVEMENT 2: Extend your arms, coming back to the starting position.

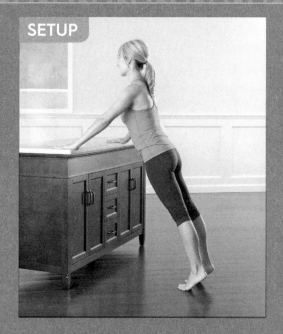

SETUP

GET DEEPER:

- Press your palms into the barre.
- Widen your shoulders down your back.
- Engage your core, keeping your hips level, and reach up through the crown of your head and down through your tailbone and heels.

MODIFICATIONS:

- To minimize discomfort in your neck or shoulders, step closer to the barre and work higher.
- To increase the intensity, do this on the floor and work on either your knees or your toes (pictured below).

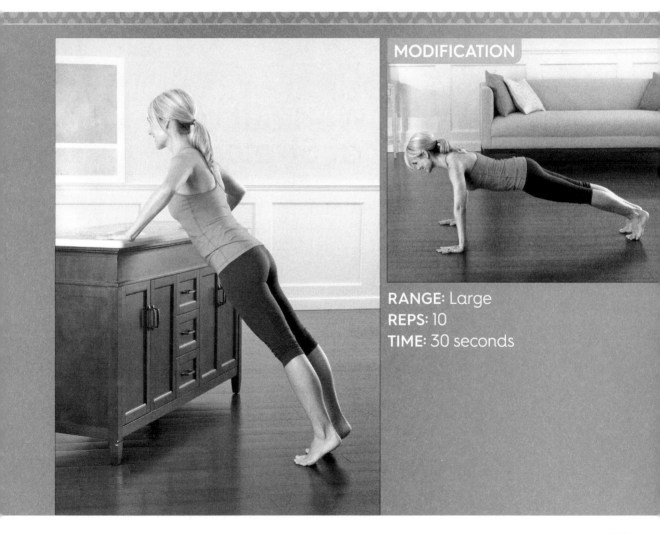

MODIFICATION

RANGE: Large
REPS: 10
TIME: 30 seconds

Week 3

LOVE YOUR LOWER BODY
Mat Workout and Mat Stretch

This week, you will add the 10-minute Love Your Lower Body Mat Workout and a 5-minute Mat Stretch to your plan. I find that working on the floor literally grounds me and helps me focus inward on my form, alignment, and breath. You have more of a foundation than just your feet on the mat—instead, you will root into your hands, knees, shins, seat, legs, and torso. This connection allows you to focus on your movement and the detail of each posture. Matwork can be more challenging than standing for some postures. Kneeling on all fours, for example, is more weight bearing than leaning against a barre. (If this creates too much pressure on your knees and shoulders, I have a great modification for you at the barre, outlined on page 173.)

This week, you'll want to begin using a yoga mat; if you don't have one, a soft surface such as a towel on carpeting can work great as well. I also recommend investing in a core ball. The ball sends you deeper into your core and glutes while supporting your neck and lower back. For years, I associated core work with crunches that left my neck burning more than my abs. Our barre3 core work using the core ball is probably the most celebrated thing among my clients—it allows them to move deeper into the muscles they want to train and relax the ones they don't. If you don't have a core ball, you can use a rolled-up towel.

Week 3

DAY 1	DAY 2	DAY 3	DAY 4	DAY 5	DAY 6	DAY 7
40 min	10 min	40 min	10 min	40 min	Rest	40 min

On Days 2 and 4, you will do the 10 Transformative Minutes.

On Days 1, 3, 4, 5, and 7, you will do the 10 Transformative Minutes, Full-Body Blast, Standing Stretch, new Mat Workout, and new Mat Stretch.

Days 1, 3, 5 & 7

10 Transformative Minutes

Horse Pose Pliés p.100

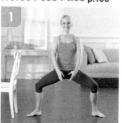

Horse Pose with Heels Lifted p.102

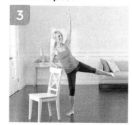

Starfish p.104

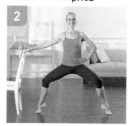

Carousel Horse p.106

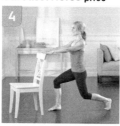

Narrow Athletic V p.108

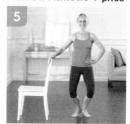

Narrow Athletic V Twists p.110

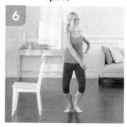

Sumo Squats p.112

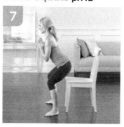

Power Leg p.114

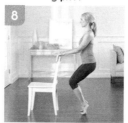

Standing Leg Lift p.116

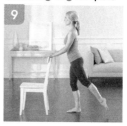

Plank p.118

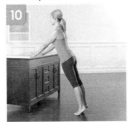

Full-Body Blast	**Horse Pose Pliés with Snow Angels** p.134	**Horse Pose with Elbow Nudges** p.136	**Starfish with Lat/Oblique Pulls** p.138

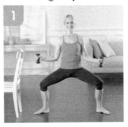

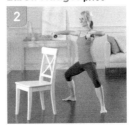

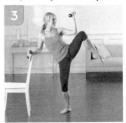

Incline Carousel Horse with Biceps Curls p.140

Incline Carousel Horse with Triceps Presses p.142

Narrow Athletic V with Rhomboid Squeezes p.144

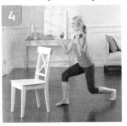

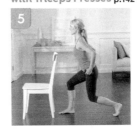

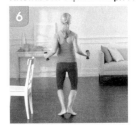

Narrow Athletic V Twists with Weights p.146

Sumo Squats with Wide Rows p.148

Power Leg with Abdominal Scoops p.150

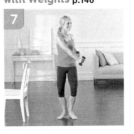

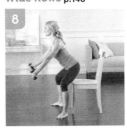

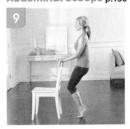

(continued)

Days 1, 3, 5 & 7 *(cont'd)*

Full-Body Blast (cont'd)

Standing Leg Lifts with Mini Triceps Pushups p.152

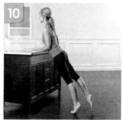
10

Wide Pushups p.154

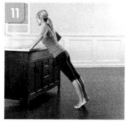
11

Standing Stretch

Triceps Foldover p.120

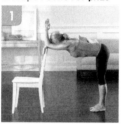
1

IT Band Stretch with a Twist p.121

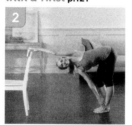
2

Crescent Lunge with Chest Opener p.122

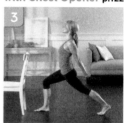
3

Heel to Seat Stretch p.123

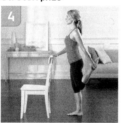
4

Figure 4 p.124

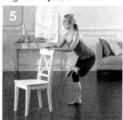
5

Mat Workout

New!

Bridge Lifts p.162

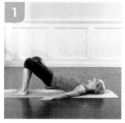
1

Bridge Lifts with Ball Hold p.164

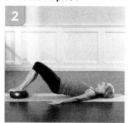
2

All Fours Levers Large p.166

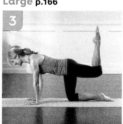
3

All Fours Levers 1 Inch p.168

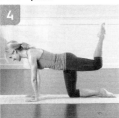

Upright Core Twists p.170

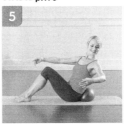

Core Rolls p.172

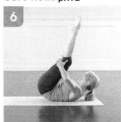

Incline Core Knee Marches p.174

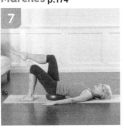

Incline Core Knee Catches p.176

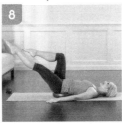

Mat Stretch

New!

Bridge Lift Hold p.178

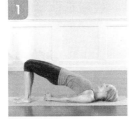

Seated Twist p.179

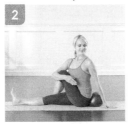

Side-Body and Inner-Thigh Stretch p.180

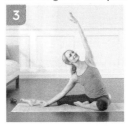

Staff Pose Deltoid Stretch p.181

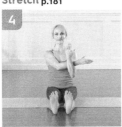

Modified Camel p.182

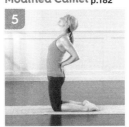

Crisscross Seated Neck Stretch p.183

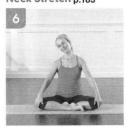

Bridge Lifts

SETUP: Lie on your back with your knees bent and your feet flat on the floor, hip-width apart. Place the core ball between your inner thighs. Open your arms a few inches away from your hips so they are in a V position with palms turned down. Your spine is in neutral. Push down with your feet and lift your hips up about 8 inches, shifting your weight to the bottoms of your shoulder blades. Hold for 5 deep breaths.

MOVEMENT 1: Lower your hips so they are hovering just above the floor.

MOVEMENT 2: Push down with your feet and lift your hips up about 8 inches, shifting your weight to the bottoms of your shoulder blades.

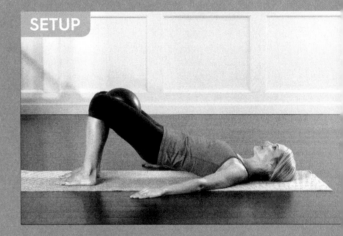

SETUP

GET DEEPER:

- Root into your feet and imagine you are dragging your heels toward your hips.
- Draw your abs in and relax your shoulders down your back.
- Squeeze the core ball between your inner thighs and engage your glutes.

MODIFICATIONS:

- To minimize lower-back or neck discomfort, keep your hips closer to the floor.
- To minimize knee discomfort, remove the core ball and open your feet wider than your hips.

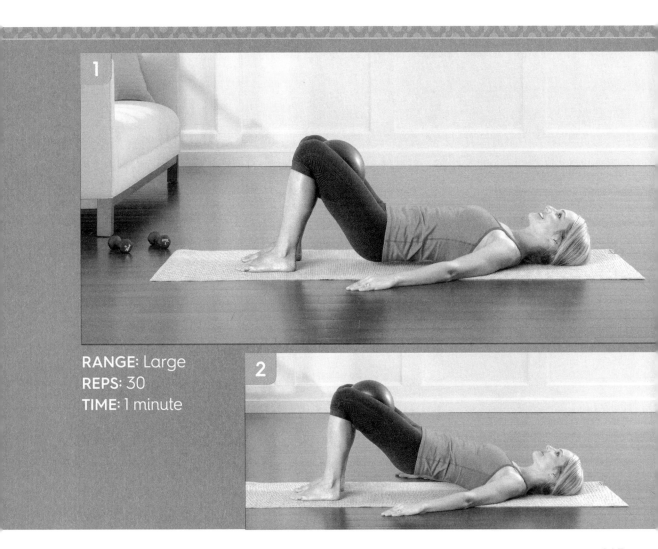

RANGE: Large
REPS: 30
TIME: 1 minute

Bridge Lifts with Ball Hold

SETUP: Lie on your back with your knees bent and your feet flat on the floor, hip-width apart. Open your arms a few inches away from your hips so they are in a V position with palms turned down. Your spine is in neutral. Place the core ball under your feet; squeeze the insides of your feet and legs together. Press your feet into the ball, lifting your hips about 2 inches off the floor but leaving your upper back and rib cage on the mat. Hold for 5 deep breaths.

MOVEMENT 1: Keep your feet pressing down into the ball as you lower your hips 1 inch.

MOVEMENT 2: Press down with your feet as you lift your hips up 1 inch.

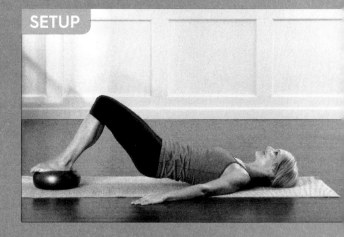

SETUP

GET DEEPER:

- Press your feet down into the core ball and squeeze your inner thighs toward each other.

- Draw your abs in and keep your upper back on the mat.

MODIFICATIONS:

- For extra stability, keep your feet flat on the floor.

- To minimize lower-back or neck discomfort, press your feet into the core ball without lifting your hips.

- For greater knee stability, place the core ball between your inner thighs.

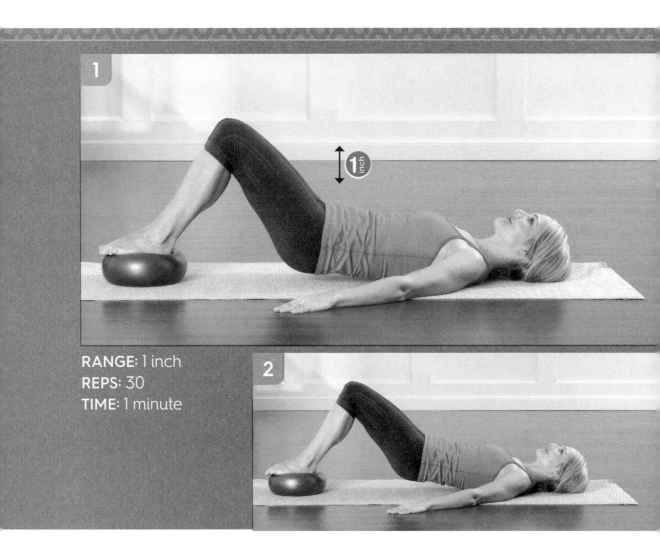

RANGE: 1 inch
REPS: 30
TIME: 1 minute

All Fours Levers Large

SETUP: Come to all fours with your hands directly under your shoulders and your knees under your hips. Draw your abs in and lengthen your lower back so your spine is long and in a neutral position. Lift your left knee to hip height and point your toes toward the ceiling. Press down with your fingers, palms, and right shin. Relax your shoulders down your back. Hold for 5 deep breaths.

MOVEMENT 1: Slowly and with control, rotate your left knee to the side without lifting your left hip.

MOVEMENT 2: Return your knee to setup position, at hip height with your toes pointing toward the ceiling.

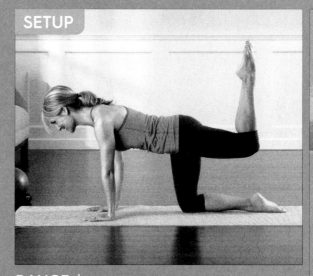

SETUP

RANGE: Large
REPS: 30 per side
TIME: 2 minutes
(1 minute per side)

GET DEEPER:

- Press into your palms evenly and widen your shoulders down your back.
- Draw your core up and in and lengthen your spine.
- Engage the side of your seat while you keep your hips steady.

MODIFICATIONS:

- To minimize knee, shoulder, or wrist discomfort, stand at the barre. Bring your feet hip-width apart, extend your right leg back, bend your knee, and fan your leg out to the side (pictured below). Work your levers from here.
- To minimize lower-back discomfort, lower your knee slightly and work smaller.
- Prop option: For more challenge and greater hamstring engagement, place the core ball behind your knee and squeeze it between your calf and hamstring.
- For a balance challenge, lift your right arm out to the side as you do your levers.

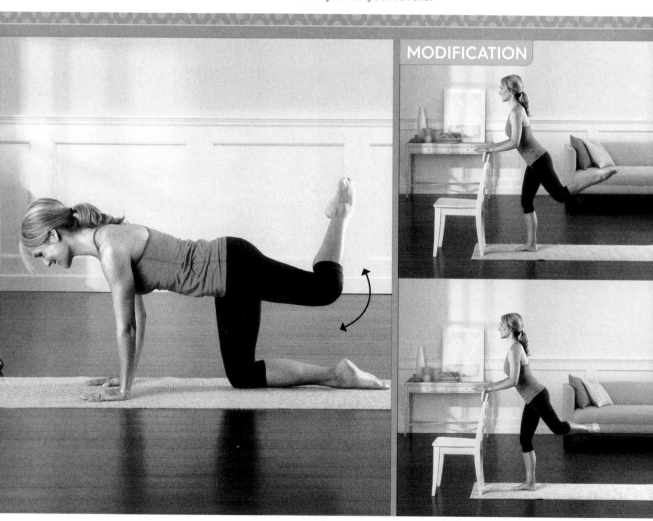

MODIFICATION

All Fours Levers 1 Inch

SETUP: Come to all fours with your hands directly under your shoulders and your knees under your hips. Draw your abs in and lengthen your lower back so your spine is long and in a neutral position. Lift your left knee to hip height and point your toes toward the ceiling. Press down with your fingers, palms, and right shin. Relax your shoulders down your back. Hold for 5 deep breaths.

MOVEMENT 1: Slowly and with control, rotate and lift your knee 1 inch.

MOVEMENT 2: Lower your knee 1 inch to return to the setup position.

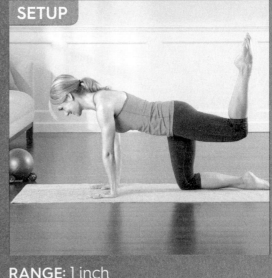

SETUP

RANGE: 1 inch
REPS: 30 per side
TIME: 2 minutes
(1 minute per side)

GET DEEPER:

- Press into your palms evenly and widen your shoulders down your back.
- Draw your core up and in and lengthen your spine.
- Engage the side of your seat while you keep your hips steady.

MODIFICATIONS:

- To minimize knee, shoulder, or wrist discomfort, stand at the barre. Bring your feet hip-width apart, extend your left leg back, bend your knee, and fan your leg out to the side (pictured below). Work your levers from here.
- To minimize lower-back discomfort, lower your knee slightly and work smaller.
- Prop option: For more challenge and greater hamstring engagement, place the core ball behind your knee and squeeze it between your calf and hamstring.
- For a balance challenge, life your right arm out to the side as you do your levers.

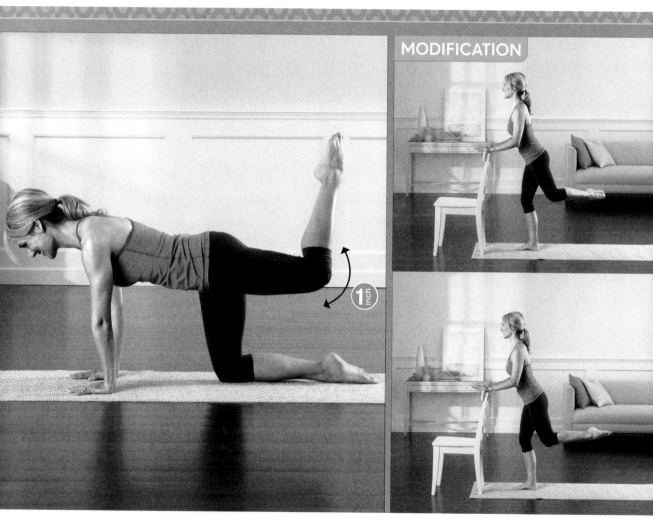

Upright Core Twists

SETUP: Sit with your core ball wedged behind your lower back, your knees bent, and your feet on the floor. Your spine is long. Draw your abs in and press your lower back into the ball. Keep your upper back lengthened and your chest open. Lift your arms in front of your shoulders and gently round them as if you were holding a beach ball. Hold for 5 deep breaths.

MOVEMENT 1: Use your core muscles to rotate your rib cage and shoulders left. Your hips stay grounded and your knees don't move. Your left arm opens to the left and your right arm stays in the starting position.

MOVEMENT 2: With control, scoop your abs as you rotate your torso back to the starting position, bringing your rib cage, shoulders, and left arm back into alignment.

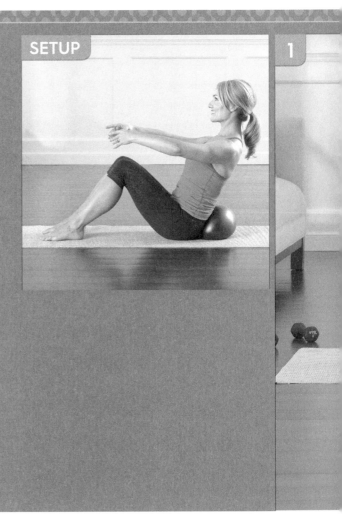

GET DEEPER:

- Keep both hips evenly weighted to the floor.
- Draw your waist in firmly.
- Inhale and exhale deeply as you twist.
- Press your back toward the core ball.

MODIFICATIONS:

- To minimize lower-back discomfort, sit more upright and move smaller.
- If you notice your hip flexors in your upper thighs engaging, extend your legs straight or bring your knees together.

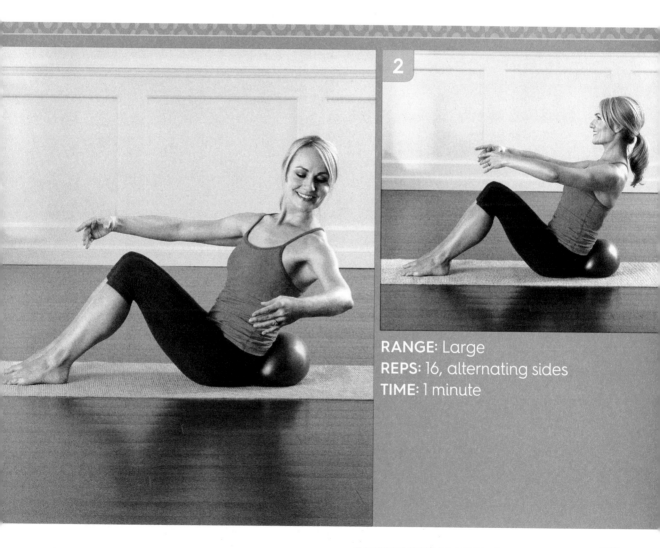

RANGE: Large
REPS: 16, alternating sides
TIME: 1 minute

Core Rolls

SETUP: Sit with your knees bent and your feet flat on the floor. Hold the backs of your thighs. Lift your feet off the ground to balance. Keep both hips weighted evenly to the floor. Draw your abs in and lift your chest. Relax your shoulders down your back. Hold for 5 deep breaths.

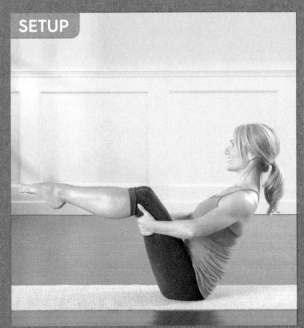

SETUP

RANGE: Large
REPS: 10
TIME: 1 minute

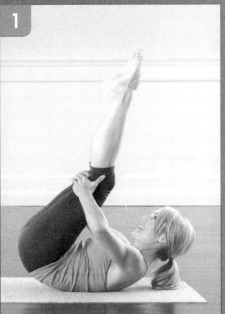

1

MOVEMENT 1: Round your back. Slowly and with control, rock back, staying in this ball-like shape. Roll only to the base of your shoulder blades, keeping a tunnel under your neck.

GET DEEPER:

- Draw your waist in and focus on moving slowly.
- Use your breath to help control your movements.

MODIFICATIONS:

- To minimize lower-back or neck discomfort, do a modified roll. Sit with the core ball wedged behind your lower back, your knees bent, and your feet on the floor. Hold the backs of your thighs. Your spine is long (pictured below). Draw your abs in to round your lower back into the ball. Keep your core engaged as you lift back to upright.
- Prop option: Place the core ball between your inner thighs and firm up and in to connect even deeper with the core.

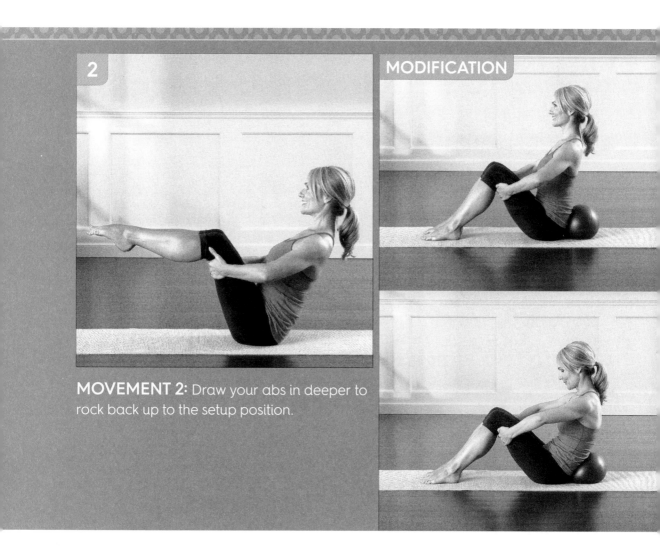

2

MOVEMENT 2: Draw your abs in deeper to rock back up to the setup position.

MODIFICATION

Incline Core Knee Marches

SETUP: Lie on your back with your knees bent and feet flat on the floor, hip-width apart. Place the core ball under your hips. Open your arms a few inches away from your hips so they are in a V position with palms turned down. Draw your abs in and lift your tailbone up slightly. Hold for 5 deep breaths.

MOVEMENT 1: Press down with your left foot as you slowly lift your right leg up to a tabletop position, knees over hips. Your right knee comes over your right hip. Your abs scoop in.

MOVEMENT 2: Slowly and with control, keep your abs drawing down toward the ball and lower your right foot to the floor.

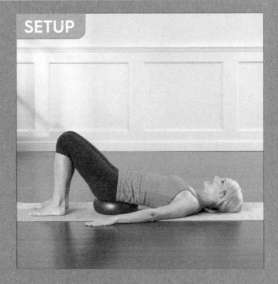

SETUP

GET DEEPER:

- Root your upper back to the floor.
- Keep your lower belly engaged and drawing inward to keep your hips still.
- Gently lift your tailbone up toward the ceiling to avoid arching over the ball.
- Engage the glutes of your supporting leg.

MODIFICATIONS:

- To minimize lower-back or neck discomfort, remove the core ball and work in a flat-back position.
- To minimize hip flexor discomfort, press the supporting foot into the floor more and don't lift your working leg as high.

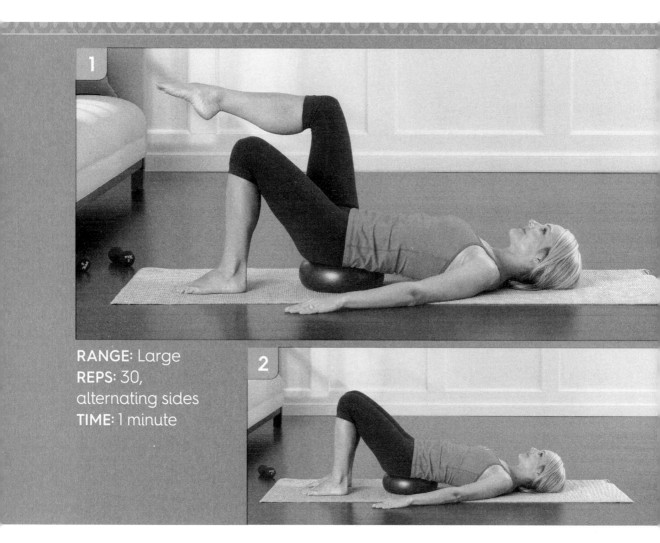

RANGE: Large
REPS: 30, alternating sides
TIME: 1 minute

Incline Core Knee Catches

SETUP: Lie on your back with your knees bent and your feet flat on the floor, hip-width apart. Place the core ball under your hips. Open your arms a few inches away from your hips so they are in a V position with palms turned down. Draw your abs in and lift your tailbone up slightly. Slowly and with control lift your right leg and then your left leg to a tabletop position, knees over hips. Hold for 5 deep breaths.

MOVEMENT 1: Keeping your abs in and hips still, straighten and extend your left leg.

MOVEMENT 2: Keeping your abs in and hips still, bend your left knee and bring your left leg back to tabletop. At the same time, straighten and extend your right leg.

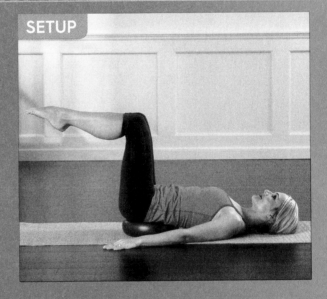

SETUP

GET DEEPER:

- Press your upper back into the floor and anchor your hips on top of the ball.
- Draw your abs in and press your rib cage into the mat.
- Relax your shoulders down your back.
- Reach your extended leg long and strong as you point your toes.

MODIFICATIONS:

- To minimize lower-back discomfort, remove the core ball and work in a flat-back position.
- To minimize hip flexor discomfort, bring your legs in closer to your chest and work smaller.
- For more stability, go slower.

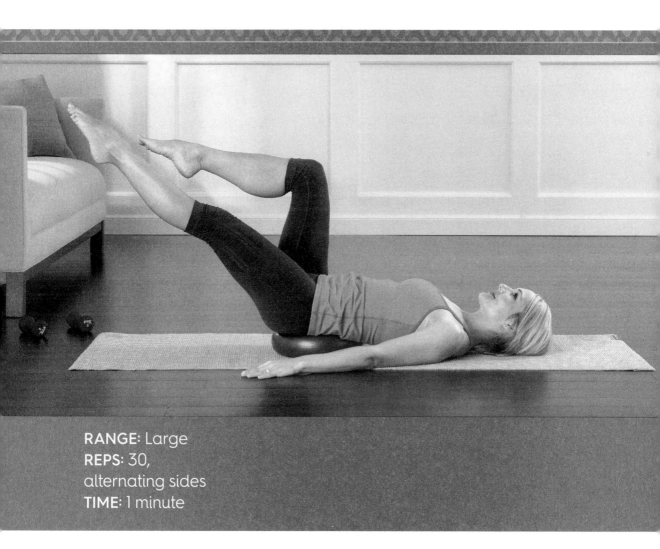

RANGE: Large
REPS: 30, alternating sides
TIME: 1 minute

Bridge Lift Hold

Lie on your back with your knees bent and your feet flat on the floor, hip-width apart. Open your arms a few inches away from your hips so they are in a V position with palms turned down. Your spine is in neutral. Push down with your feet and lift your hips up about 8 inches, shifting your weight to the bottom of your shoulder blades. Interlace your fingers behind your back. Reach your hands toward your ankles and press the sides of your arms and your feet down. Lift up with your hips, belly, and chest. Hold for 5 deep breaths.

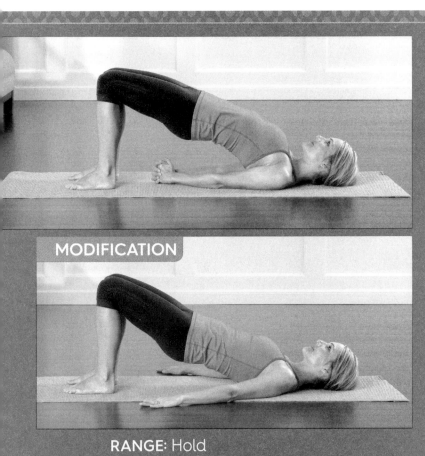

MODIFICATION

RANGE: Hold
REPS: 1
TIME: 30 seconds

GET DEEPER:

- **Press firmly through your feet to engage your hamstrings and glutes.**

- **Keep your knees hip-width apart by gently engaging your inner thighs—don't let your knees drift to the sides. Expand your belly and chest toward the ceiling.**

MODIFICATIONS:

- **To minimize shoulder or neck discomfort, keep your hands in a low V at your sides (pictured left).**

- **To minimize knee discomfort, walk your feet wider than hip width or place the core ball between your inner thighs.**

Seated Twist

Sit with your spine long and your legs extended in front of you. Bend your left knee toward the ceiling, placing your left foot outside of your right knee. Twist at your waist to the left, turning your rib cage and shoulders and wrapping your right arm around your left knee. Place your left hand on the floor behind you to help you stay balanced. Hold for 5 deep breaths, then switch sides.

GET DEEPER:

- **Keep your hips level and hug your knee in tight.**
- **On your inhales, lengthen your spine.**
- **On your exhales, deepen your twist.**
- **Firm your lower belly in.**
- **Relax your shoulders down your back.**

MODIFICATIONS:

- **Prop option: Wedge the core ball behind your hips to support the body with a neutral spine.**

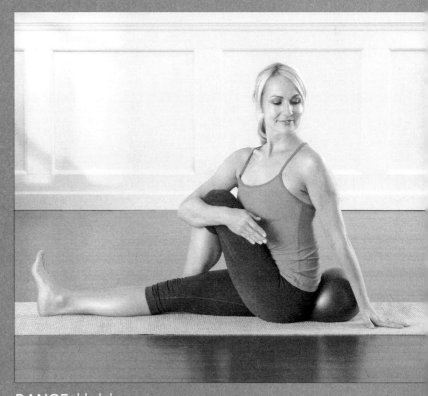

RANGE: Hold
REPS: 1 per side
TIME: 1 minute
(30 seconds per side)

Side-Body and Inner-Thigh Stretch

Sit with your spine long and your right leg extended to the side, toes pointed. Bring the sole of your left foot to your right inner thigh. Place your right hand on the floor inside your right leg. Reach your left arm overhead; lean up and over the extended leg in a side-body stretch. Keep both hips rooted to the floor evenly. Hold for 5 deep breaths, then switch sides.

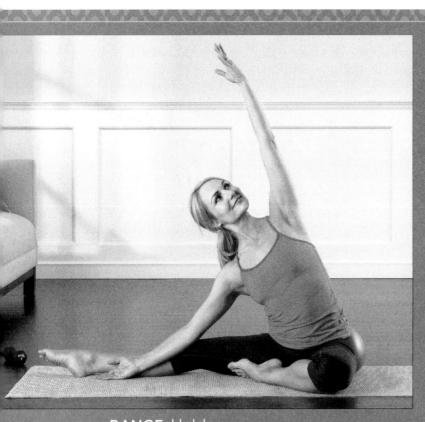

GET DEEPER:

- Lengthen the side body and arm. Engage your core.
- Point your toes and root both legs down to the floor.
- Keep your shoulders wide and down your back.

MODIFICATIONS:

- To minimize lower-back discomfort, work higher.
- Prop option: Wedge the core ball behind your hips to support the body with a neutral spine.

RANGE: Hold
REP: 1 per side
TIME: 1 minute
(30 seconds per side)

Staff Pose Deltoid Stretch

Sit with your spine long and your legs extended in front of you, feet flexed. Reach your right arm across your chest. Use your left arm to pull your right arm closer to your body. Keep your spine long as you gently hinge forward, stretching the backs of your legs. Hold for 5 deep breaths, then switch sides.

GET DEEPER:

- **Press your legs down.**
- **Relax your shoulders down your back.**
- **Lengthen your spine as you firm your core in.**

MODIFICATIONS:

- **For tight hamstrings, bend your knees slightly.**
- **Prop option: Wedge the core ball behind your hips to support your body with a neutral spine.**

RANGE: Hold
REPS: 1 per side
TIME: 1 minute
(30 seconds per side)

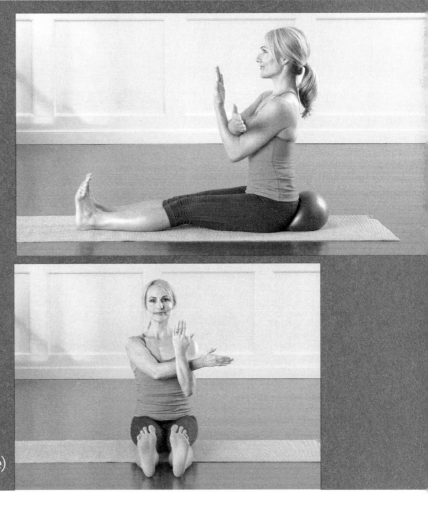

Modified Camel

Kneel with your shins hip-width apart. Your shoulders, hips, and knees are in one straight line. Bring your hands to your lower back with your fingers pointing toward the floor and your elbows back behind you. Slowly and with control, move into a small backward bend by pushing your hips, belly, and chest forward. Lift your head back as you gaze up the wall and toward the ceiling. Hold for 5 deep breaths.

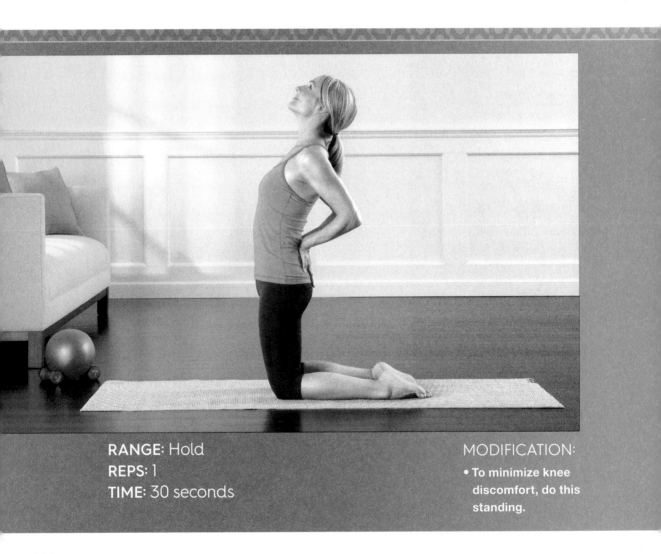

RANGE: Hold
REPS: 1
TIME: 30 seconds

MODIFICATION:
• To minimize knee discomfort, do this standing.

Crisscross Seated Neck Stretch

Sit with your spine long and your legs crossed in front of you. Open your arms to form a low V with your fingers brushing the floor. Lower your chin toward your chest, then roll your right ear over your right shoulder. Reach long through your left fingertips. Hold for 5 deep breaths, then switch sides.

GET DEEPER:

- **Press your hips into the floor and draw your abs in.**
- **Relax your shoulders down your back and lengthen your spine.**
- **Gently extend your arm to the side.**

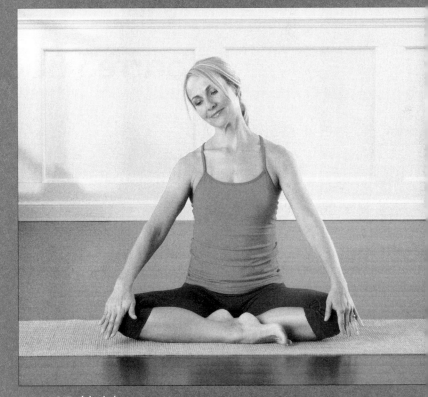

RANGE: Hold
REPS: 1 per side
TIME: 1 minute (30 seconds per side)

Week 4

barre3 Boost #1

Are you ready to increase your productivity this week? Get ready to move all day and take your practice to the next level. This week, I introduce barre3 Boosts. Barre3 Boosts are 1- to 5-minute full-body workouts that you can do anytime to get a quick burst of energy.

As you learned in Chapter 2, getting up and moving all day long is good for your health and for your waistline. The barre3 Boosts are perfect moves to do throughout the day when you start to feel antsy after sitting too long or when you need a pick-me-up. These short exercise segments are designed to boost your heart rate—and with it your calorie burn—all in even less time than a traditional Love Your Lower Body routine.

In addition to these boosts, this week you will focus on spreading out your activity during the day by doing a series of 10-minute workouts. To indicate how to break up the workouts as the day goes on, look for the following cues: Morning Wake-Up, Power Lunch, Late-Afternoon Metabolic Boost, and Evening Express. While you may not be able to work out in 10-minute bursts four times a day every day, I ask that you trust the process and give this your very best shot. If you're having a hard time staying on track, keep in mind that 10 minutes isn't a big time commitment—and it's just enough time to boost your energy and refocus your mind while you're answering e-mails, sitting on hold with tech support, or taking a little break from chores.

Turn the page for your workout at a glance.

Week 4

DAY 1	DAY 2	DAY 3	DAY 4	DAY 5	DAY 6	DAY 7
40 min	10 min	40 min	10 min	40 min	Rest	40 min

On Days 2 and 4, you will do the 10 Transformative Minutes.

On Days 1, 3, 5, and 7, you will do the new barre3 Boost #1, 10 Transformative Minutes, Full-Body Blast, Mat Workout, and Stretch.

Days 1, 3, 5 & 7

barre3 Boost #1

New!

Morning Wake-Up:

Wake up with your new barre3 Boost (5 minutes).

Push-Pulls p.190

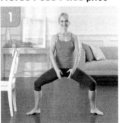

Crescent Lunge with Chest Opener p.122

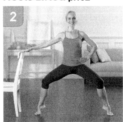

New! Hold for 1 min per side

---

10 Transformative Minutes

Power Lunch:

Before lunch, squeeze in the 10 Transformative Minutes (10 minutes).

Horse Pose Pliés p.100

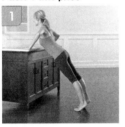

Horse Pose with Heels Lifted p.102

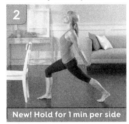

Starfish p.104

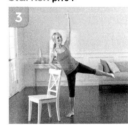

Carousel Horse p.106

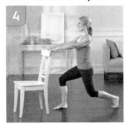

Narrow Athletic V p.108

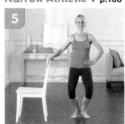

Narrow Athletic V Twists p.110

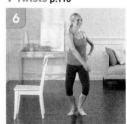

Sumo Squats p.112

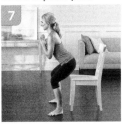

Power Leg p.114

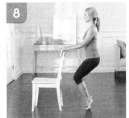

Standing Leg Lift p.116

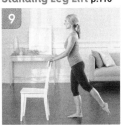

Plank p.118

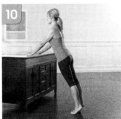

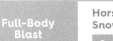
Full-Body Blast

Late-Afternoon Metabolic Boost:

To fight the late-afternoon slump, grab your weights and do the Full-Body Blast (10 minutes).

Horse Pose Pliés with Snow Angels p.134

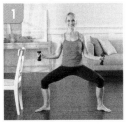

Horse Pose with Elbow Nudges p.136

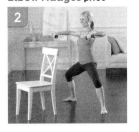

Starfish with Lat/Oblique Pulls p.138

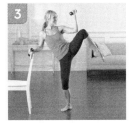

Incline Carousel Horse with Biceps Curls p.140

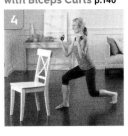

Incline Carousel Horse with Triceps Presses p.142

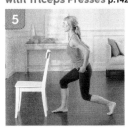

Narrow Athletic V with Rhomboid Squeezes p.144

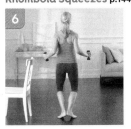

(continued)

Days 1, 3, 5 & 7 *(cont'd)*

Full-Body Blast *(cont'd)*

Narrow Athletic V Twists with Weights p.146

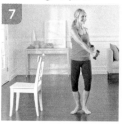

Sumo Squats with Wide Rows p.148

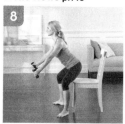

Power Leg with Abdominal Scoops p.150

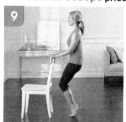

Standing Leg Lifts with Mini Triceps Pushups p.152

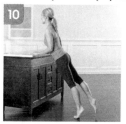

Wide Pushups p.154

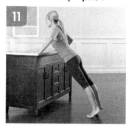

Mat Workout

Evening Express:

As your day winds down, find a quiet corner and do the Mat Workout and Mat Stretch (10 minutes).

Bridge Lifts p.162

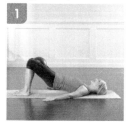

Bridge Lifts with Ball Hold p.164

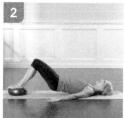

All Fours Levers Large p.166

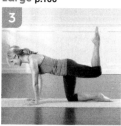

All Fours Levers 1 Inch p.168

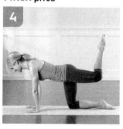

Upright Core Twists p.170

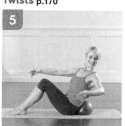

Core Rolls p.172

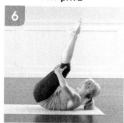

Incline Core Knee Marches p.174

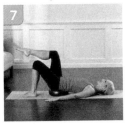

Incline Core Knee Catches p.176

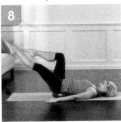

Mat Stretch

Bridge Lift Hold p.178

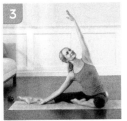

Seated Twist p.179

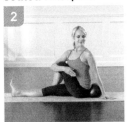

Side-Body and Inner-Thigh Stretch p.180

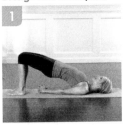

Staff Pose Deltoid Stretch p.181

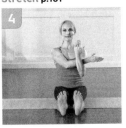

Modified Camel p.182

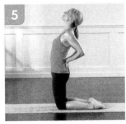

Crisscross Seated Neck Stretch p.183

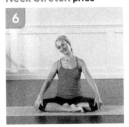

Push-Pulls

SETUP: Place your palms wider than your shoulders on the barre. Walk your feet back and bend at your waist so your feet are underneath your hips and your arms and back are straight (your body makes an L shape). Press down with your feet, gently bend your knees, draw your abs in, and lengthen your spine. Hold for 5 deep breaths.

Do these on a sturdy surface like a wall-mounted counter or kitchen island.

MOVEMENT 1: Lift your heels and rise up to Plank position. Continue to press your hands into the barre. Your ears, shoulders, hips, and heels should be in line and your spine neutral. Relax your shoulders down your back.

MOVEMENT 2: Bend your elbows to lower into a pushup position. Your elbows stay in line with your wrists and your body stays in one long line from your heels to your head.

MOVEMENT 3: Straighten your arms to come back to Plank position. Pull your hips back over your heels, bringing your body back to the L-shape setup position.

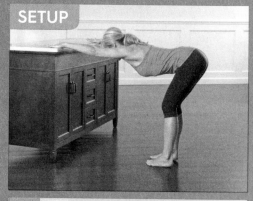

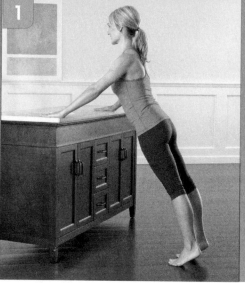

GET DEEPER:

- Press your palms down on the barre.
- Draw your core in and keep your hips level.
- Reach up through the crown of your head and down with your heels.
- Firm your core in as you lower into your pushup.
- Pull your hips back over your heels in the L shape and keep your shoulders wide and down your back.

MODIFICATION:

- To minimize wrist, neck, or shoulder discomfort, step closer to the barre and keep your pushup higher.
- Prop option: Place the core ball between your inner thighs to engage your core more deeply.
- Bend your knees as much as needed to make your spine long when you are bent over in the L shape.

Push-Pulls are made up of moves you have already learned. However, in this exercise, I sequence the movements so they have a continuous flow. Push-Pulls are a signature barre3 exercise we do in every class because they strategically strengthen, lengthen, and burn calories in a short amount of time.

RANGE: Large
REPS: Varies; repeat for 3 minutes.
TIME: 3 minutes

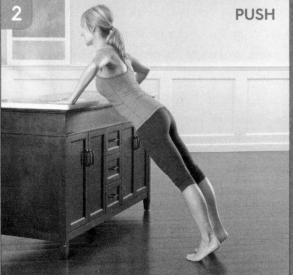

2   PUSH

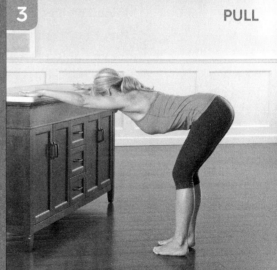

3   PULL

Week 5

barre3 Boosts
#2 and #3

This week, I have outlined two paths to choose from. You can do a 40-minute continuous sequence (Path 1) or break the 40 minutes of exercise up into mini-routines you do throughout the day (Path 2). Moving through four workouts without a break can be challenging. I find that on days when I'm low on energy, the only workout I can imagine doing is a short one. I usually start out planning to do just 10 minutes of exercise, but often after finishing that segment, I want to keep moving. I didn't set out with the intention of moving for 40 minutes, but once I started, I wasn't ready to stop! Try it. If you don't want to keep going, plan to pick up the other workouts later on in the day.

My goal for you is to make these workouts your own. Finding your natural rhythm will help make exercise an integrated and valued part of your life. Timing isn't the only way to personalize this program: You can also try the different modifications to mold these moves to fit your lifestyle and body. If you simply can't find a modification that works for you, swap out the full move and replace it with an exercise you can do that works similar body parts. For example, if working on your toes in Power Leg doesn't feel good on your feet but you love Sumo Squats, feel free to substitute in Sumo Squats. You can also substitute entire 10-minute workouts! If you're traveling, you may want to skip the Mat Workout and move through the 10 Transformative Minutes instead. As you progress through Weeks 6, 7, and 8 of the program, I'll continue to teach you new ways to combine workouts and get deeper into your moves—but there's plenty of room for you to get creative when it comes to making this program really work for you.

This same philosophy applies to what you are serving up on your plate. For the past month, you have learned the power of combining healthy proteins, fats, and fiber at each and every meal. You have likely experimented with substituting ingredients or even making your own creations. I encourage you to continue. Use the recipes in Chapter 7 as a foundation for your own inventions. My favorite recipes in this whole bunch are the DIY smoothies, salads, and bowls because there are endless (and easy) ways to re-create them while sticking to this plan. When you eat out, see if you can have the kitchen modify meals to meet our guidelines. I have learned to quickly scan the menu for veggie sides and main courses that have grilled fish and meat.

At the end of these 8 weeks, I want you to have the tools to look at a menu, the contents in your fridge, or the selections at your salad bar and quickly make a choice that is balanced and designed to both nourish you and fuel your weight-loss goals.

Week 5

DAY 1	DAY 2	DAY 3	DAY 4	DAY 5	DAY 6	DAY 7
40 min	10 min	40 min	10 min	40 min	Rest	40 min

On Days 2 and 4, you will do the 10 Transformative Minutes.

On Days 1, 3, 5, and 7, you will do the Standing Stretch, the new barre3 Boost #2, the Full-Body Blast, the new barre3 Boost #3, the Mat Workout, and the Mat Stretch. You can do your workouts in one 40-minute training session or break them up throughout the day with the suggestions below.

Days 1, 3, 5 & 7

Standing Stretch

Morning Wake-Up:

Enjoy your Standing Stretch and wake up with your new barre3 Boost #2 (10 minutes).

Triceps Foldover p.120

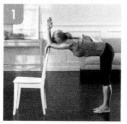

IT Band Stretch with a Twist p.121

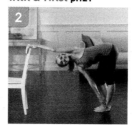

Crescent Lunge with Chest Opener p.122

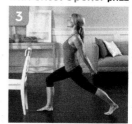

Heel to Seat Stretch p.123

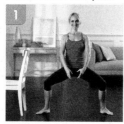

Figure 4 p.124

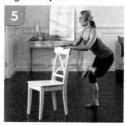

barre3 Boost #2

New!

Horse Pose Pliés p.100

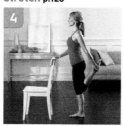

Sumo Squats p.112

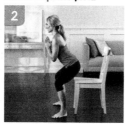

Push-Pulls p.190

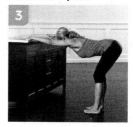

Midmorning Energizer:

Keep your metabolism revving midmorning with the Full-Body Blast (10 minutes).

Horse Pose Pliés with Snow Angels p.134

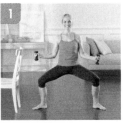

Horse Pose with Elbow Nudges p.136

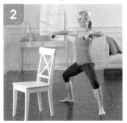

Starfish with Lat/Oblique Pulls p.138

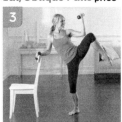

Incline Carousel Horse with Biceps Curls p.140

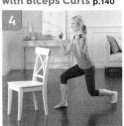

Incline Carousel Horse with Triceps Presses p.142

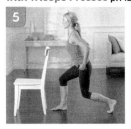

Narrow Athletic V with Rhomboid Squeezes p.144

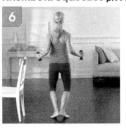

Narrow Athletic V Twists with Weights p.146

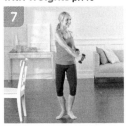

Sumo Squats with Wide Rows p.148

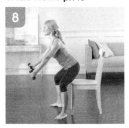

Power Leg with Abdominal Scoops p.150

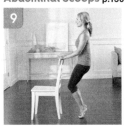

Standing Leg Lifts with Mini Triceps Pushups p.152

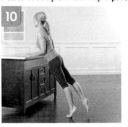

Wide Pushups p.154

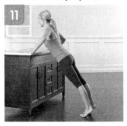

(continued)

| barre3 Boost #3 | Horse Pose Pliés **p.100** | Starfish **p.138** | Incline Core Knee Catches **p.176** |

New!

Power Lunch:

Do the new barre3 Boost #3 twice on your lunch break (5 minutes).

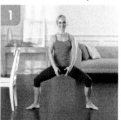
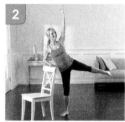
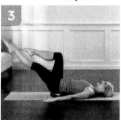

| Mat Workout | Bridge Lifts **p.162** | Bridge Lifts with Ball Hold **p.164** | All Fours Levers Large **p.166** |

Late-Afternoon Metabolic Boost:

Grab your yoga mat and clear your mind with the Mat Workout (10 minutes).

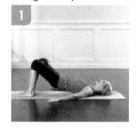
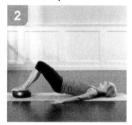
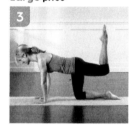

All Fours Levers 1 Inch **p.168**   Upright Core Twists **p.170**   Core Rolls **p.172**

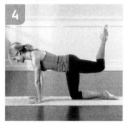
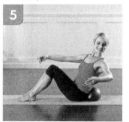
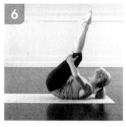

Incline Core Knee Marches **p.174**   Incline Core Knee Catches **p.176**

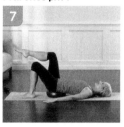
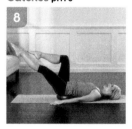

Mat Stretch

Evening Express:

Before getting into bed, calm your mind and lengthen your body with the Mat Stretch (5 minutes).

Bridge Lift Hold p.178

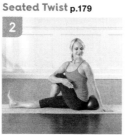

Seated Twist p.179

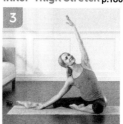

Side-Body and Inner-Thigh Stretch p.180

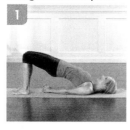

Staff Pose Deltoid Stretch p.181

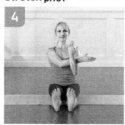

Modified Camel p.182

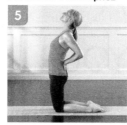

Crisscross Seated Neck Stretch p.183

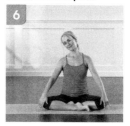

Week 6

LOVE YOUR LOWER BODY
Glute Combo Workout

At this point, you have mastered the art of coaxing the very most out of each posture. Now it is time to focus on areas of the body that need extra attention—starting with the glutes. Most of my clients have weak glutes but strong quads. This is partly a symptom of a modern, sedentary lifestyle: We use our quads to walk and to climb stairs, but our glutes aren't as engaged during day-to-day life. When we sit, our quads get shorter and our glutes get stretched out, which is also problematic. These imbalances can lead to myriad health issues, including lower-back pain. To bring your body into balance, I've created a 10-minute Glute Combo Workout designed to shape and lift your seat. But don't worry, you won't need to learn new moves. I have strategically sequenced the very best of our glute exercises from previous Love Your Lower Body workouts into one highly targeted butt-burner. By strengthening the muscles in your seat, you'll reduce lower-back pain while shaping and tightening your entire lower body.

The workout path for this week begins with your new Glute Combo Workout, followed by a 30-minute workout later in the day. Feel free do those 30 minutes continuously or broken into short 10-minute workouts.

Week 6

DAY 1	DAY 2	DAY 3	DAY 4	DAY 5	DAY 6	DAY 7
40 min	10 min	40 min	10 min	40 min	Rest	40 min

On Days 2 and 4, you will do the 10 Transformative Minutes.

On Days 1, 3, 5, and 7, you will do the new Glute Combo Workout in the morning, followed later in the day by the 10 Transformative Minutes, the Standing Stretch, the Mat Workout, and the Mat Stretch.

Days 1, 3, 5 & 7

Glute Combo Workout

New!

Sumo Squats p.112

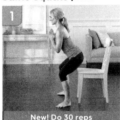

New! Do 30 reps

Narrow Athletic V p.108

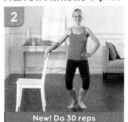

New! Do 30 reps

Standing Leg Lifts p.116

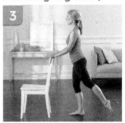

All Fours Levers Large p.166

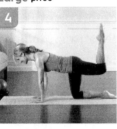

Bridge Lifts p.162

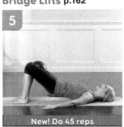

New! Do 45 reps

Bridge Lifts with Ball Hold p.164

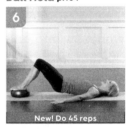

New! Do 45 reps

Seated Twist p.179

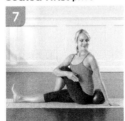

10 Transformative Minutes

Horse Pose Pliés p.100

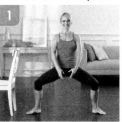

Horse Pose with Heels Lifted p.102

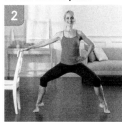

Starfish p.104

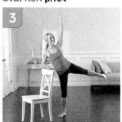

Carousel Horse p.106

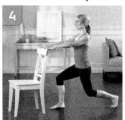

Narrow Athletic V p.108

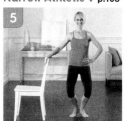

Narrow Athletic V Twists p.110

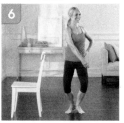

Sumo Squats p.112

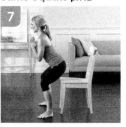

Power Leg p.114

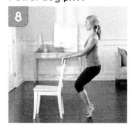

Standing Leg Lift p.116

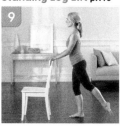

Plank p.118

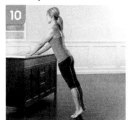

(continued)

Days 1, 3, 5 & 7 *(cont'd)*

Standing Stretch

Triceps Foldover p.120

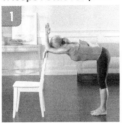

IT Band Stretch with a Twist p.121

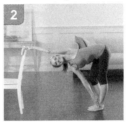

Crescent Lunge with Chest Opener p.122

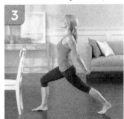

Heel to Seat Stretch p.123

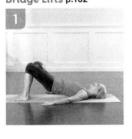

Figure 4 p.124

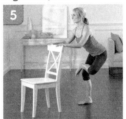

Mat Workout

Bridge Lifts p.162

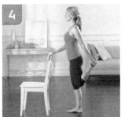

Bridge Lifts with Ball Hold p.164

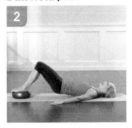

All Fours Levers Large p.166

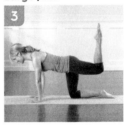

All Fours Levers 1 Inch p.168

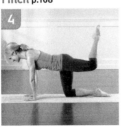

Upright Core Twists p.170

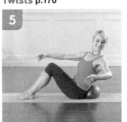

Core Rolls p.172

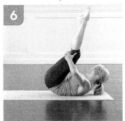

Incline Core Knee Marches p.174

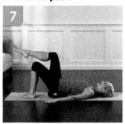

Incline Core Knee Catches p.176

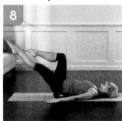

Mat Stretch

Bridge Lift Hold p.178

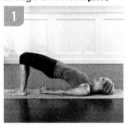

Seated Twist p.179

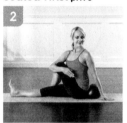

Side-Body and Inner-Thigh Stretch p.180

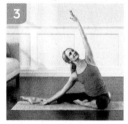

Staff Pose Deltoid Stretch p.181

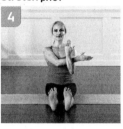

Modified Camel p.182

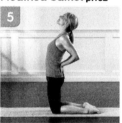

Crisscross Seated Neck Stretch p.183

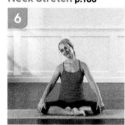

Week 7

LOVE YOUR LOWER BODY
Core Combo Workout

Last week, we targeted the glutes. This week, we go deep with a new workout designed to strengthen your core. It's made up of my favorite Love Your Lower Body moves. You will notice that the first half of the workout is standing. I'm a big fan of standing core work, because it trains your body to stand tall as you work toward a strong, lean midsection.

Barre3's core values are about a whole lot more than flat abs. They really focus on the connection between food and exercise. The recipes in this plan are literally designed to support your deep core—your gut. The intestines play a big role in how we process food, both in burning calories to lose weight and in absorbing nutrients to gain energy. The foods on this plan are easy on the gut and will ultimately help you trim your waistline and flatten your tummy.

The workout path for this week begins with your new Core Combo Workout, followed by a 30-minute workout later in the day. Feel free do those 30 minutes continuously or broken into short 10-minute workouts.

Week 7

DAY 1	DAY 2	DAY 3	DAY 4	DAY 5	DAY 6	DAY 7
40 min	10 min	40 min	10 min	40 min	Rest	40 min

On Days 2 and 4, you will do the 10 Transformative Minutes.

On Days 1, 3, 5, and 7, you will do the new Core Combo Workout in the morning, followed later in the day by the Full-Body Blast, the Standing Stretch, the Mat Workout, and the Mat Stretch.

Days 1, 3, 5 & 7

Core Combo Workout

New!

Horse Pose Pliés p.100

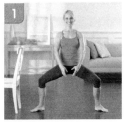

Starfish with Lat/Oblique Pulls p.138

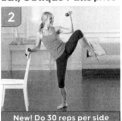

New! Do 30 reps per side

Plank (at the barre) p.118

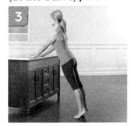

Plank (on the floor) p.119

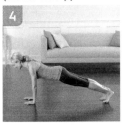

Upright Core Twists p.170

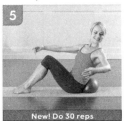

New! Do 30 reps

Core Rolls p.172

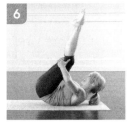

Incline Core Knee Marches p.174

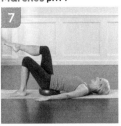

Incline Core Knee Catches p.176

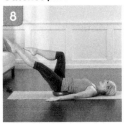

Bridge Lifts with Ball Hold p.164

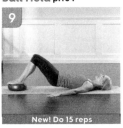

New! Do 15 reps

Full-Body Blast

Midmorning Energizer:

Keep your metabolism revving midmorning with the Full-Body Blast (10 minutes).

Horse Pose Pliés with Snow Angels p.134

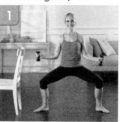

Horse Pose with Elbow Nudges p.136

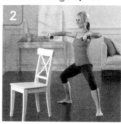

Starfish with Lat/Oblique Pulls p.138

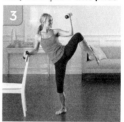

Incline Carousel Horse with Biceps Curls p.140

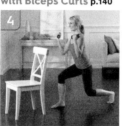

Incline Carousel Horse with Triceps Presses p.142

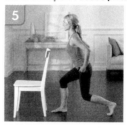

Narrow Athletic V with Rhomboid Squeezes p.144

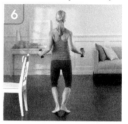

Narrow Athletic V Twists with Weights p.146

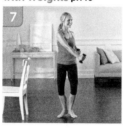

Sumo Squats with Wide Rows p.148

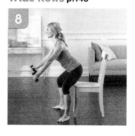

Power Leg with Abdominal Scoops p.150

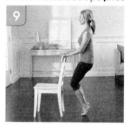

Standing Leg Lifts with Mini Triceps Pushups p.152

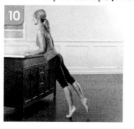

Wide Pushups p.165

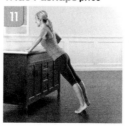

(continued)

Days 1, 3, 5 & 7 *(cont'd)*

Standing Stretch

Triceps Foldover p.120
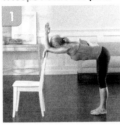

IT Band Stretch with a Twist p.121
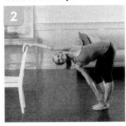

Crescent Lunge with Chest Opener p.122
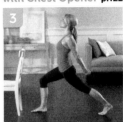

Heel to Seat Stretch p.123
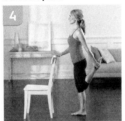

Figure 4 p.124
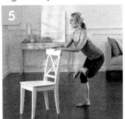

Mat Workout

Bridge Lifts p.162
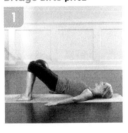

Bridge Lifts with Ball Hold p.164
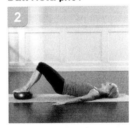

All Fours Levers Large p.166
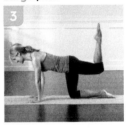

All Fours Levers 1 Inch p.168
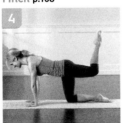

Upright Core Twists p.170
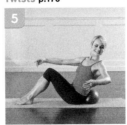

Core Rolls p.172
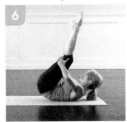

Incline Core Knee Marches p.174

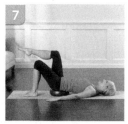

Incline Core Knee Catches p.176

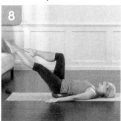

Mat Stretch

Bridge Lift Hold p.178

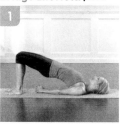

Seated Twist p.179

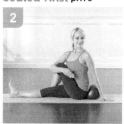

Side-Body and Inner-Thigh Stretch p.180

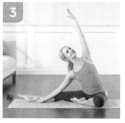

Staff Pose Deltoid Stretch p.181

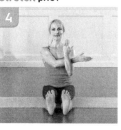

Modified Camel p.182

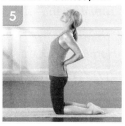

Crisscross Seated Neck Stretch p.183

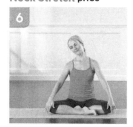

Week 8

Fully Commit

Before launching into your 8th week, take a moment to reflect on your progress so far. If you are like the women who tested this program with me, you've had good days and not-so-good days. You have taken great liberties in "making it your own." You have discovered that some of the exercises are easier for you to do, while you avoid others altogether. You may have latched on to a couple of key recipes, making them more than once, and skipped others that sounded unappealing. You probably had a hard time eliminating sugar—including alcohol—so you found ways to rationalize in the name of being "balanced." I know this, because I do the same thing! It's okay, we are all human, and I believe in moderation and balance. That being said, this is your week to fully commit.

Are you ready to take your results to the next level? Even if you fell off the wagon for a few days (or weeks), I believe you will be amazed—and probably a little surprised—at the results you get. If you decided to keep your double skinny vanilla latte and muffin over the past 7 weeks, this is your week to swap in a smoothie or another barre3-balanced breakfast at home. If you have taken a liking to working out only 10 minutes a day, this is your week to push yourself and do 30 or 40 minutes in a day. If you have skipped out on catching your z's, this is your week to do whatever you must to get your 8 hours. If you have shied away from reaching out and sharing your program with friends and family, this is your week to commit publicly and gather support. Better yet, find a friend to join you and finish off strong with her by your side.

One of my favorite expressions is "It's the sand in the oyster that makes the pearl." Making yourself a little uncomfortable can lead to amazing transformation. When your muscles are sore and pushed to their limits, it's because they are building greater strength. Embrace the idea of pushing yourself out of your comfort zone and really make this last week of the program your strongest and most committed yet.

This week you'll work both the Glute Combo and the Core Combo into your routine, doing one of them in the morning, followed by a 30-minute workout later in the day. Just as in the past 2 weeks, you can choose to break those workouts up or do them together.

Week 8

DAY 1	DAY 2	DAY 3	DAY 4	DAY 5	DAY 6	DAY 7
40 min	10 min	40 min	10 min	40 min	Rest	40 min

On Days 2 and 4, you will do the 10 Transformative Minutes.

On Days 1 and 3, you will do the Core Combo Workout, the 10 Transformative Minutes, the Standing Stretch, the Mat Workout, and the Mat Stretch.

On Days 5 and 7, you will do the Glute Combo Workout, the 10 Transformative Minutes, the Standing Stretch, the Mat Workout, and the Mat Stretch.

Additionally, on Days 1 through 7, do one of the barre3 Boosts in the sidebar "Move All Day!" on page 219 to get up and move for 1 minute.

Days 1 & 3

Core Combo Workout

Horse Pose Pliés p.100

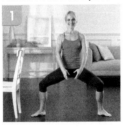

Starfish with Lat/Oblique Pulls p.138

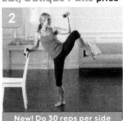

New! Do 30 reps per side

Plank (at the barre) p.118

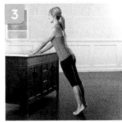

Plank (on the floor) p.119

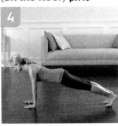

Upright Core Twists p.170

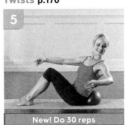

New! Do 30 reps

Core Rolls p.172

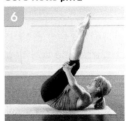

Incline Core Knee Marches p.174

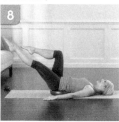

7

Incline Core Knee Catches p.176

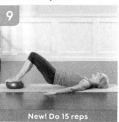

8

Bridge Lifts with Ball Hold p.164

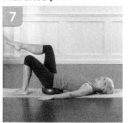

9

New! Do 15 reps

10 Transformative Minutes

Horse Pose Pliés p.100

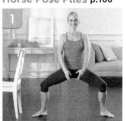

1

Horse Pose with Heels Lifted p.102

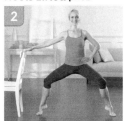

2

Starfish p.104

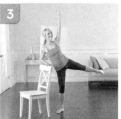

3

Carousel Horse p.106

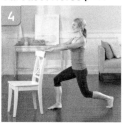

4

Narrow Athletic V p.108

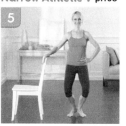

5

Narrow Athletic V Twists p.110

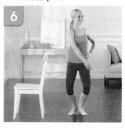

6

Sumo Squats p.112

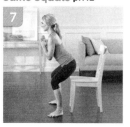

7

Power Leg p.114

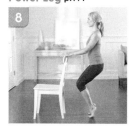

8

Standing Leg Lift p.116

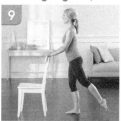

9

(continued)

Days 1 & 3 *(cont'd)*

**10
Transformative
Minutes
(cont'd)**

Plank p.118

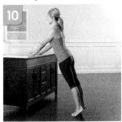

**Standing
Stretch**

Triceps Foldover p.120

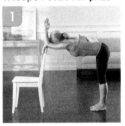

**IT Band Stretch
with a Twist p.121**

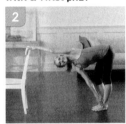

**Crescent Lunge
with Chest Opener p.122**

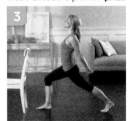

**Heel to Seat
Stretch p.123**

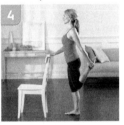

Figure 4 p.124

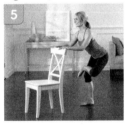

**Mat
Workout**

Bridge Lifts p.162

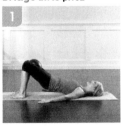

**Bridge Lifts with
Ball Hold p.164**

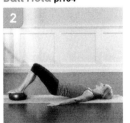

**All Fours Levers
Large p.166**

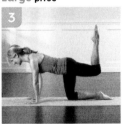

All Fours Levers 1 Inch **p.168**

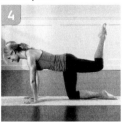

Upright Core Twists **p.170**

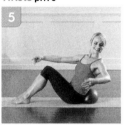

Core Rolls **p.172**

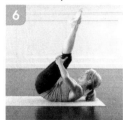

Incline Core Knee Marches **p.174**

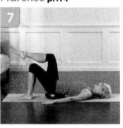

Incline Core Knee Catches **p.176**

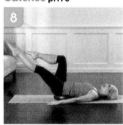

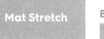

Mat Stretch

Bridge Lift Hold **p.178**

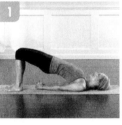

Seated Twist **p.179**

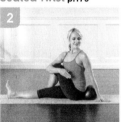

Side-Body and Inner-Thigh Stretch **p.180**

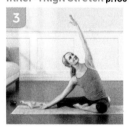

Staff Pose Deltoid Stretch **p.181**

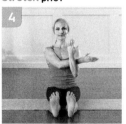

Modified Camel **p.182**

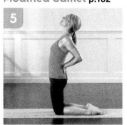

Crisscross Seated Neck Stretch **p.183**

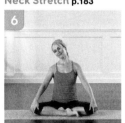

(continued)

Days 5 & 7

Glute Combo Workout

Sumo Squats p.112

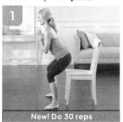

New! Do 30 reps

Narrow Athletic V p.108

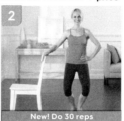

New! Do 30 reps

Standing Leg Lifts p.116

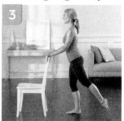

All Fours Levers Large p.166

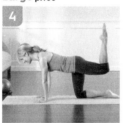

Bridge Lifts p.162

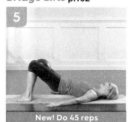

New! Do 45 reps

Bridge Lifts with Ball Hold p.164

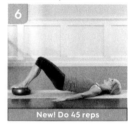

New! Do 45 reps

Seated Twist p.179

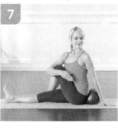

10 Transformative Minutes

Horse Pose Pliés p.100

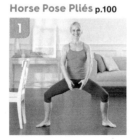

Horse Pose with Heels Lifted p.102

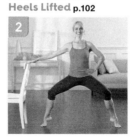

Starfish p.104

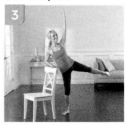

Carousel Horse p.106

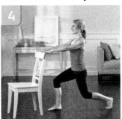

Narrow Athletic V p.108

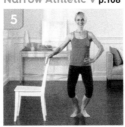

Narrow Athletic V Twists p.110

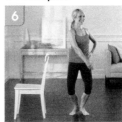

Sumo Squats p.112

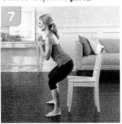

Power Leg p.114

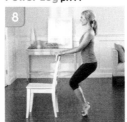

Standing Leg Lift p.116

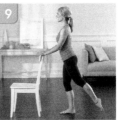

Plank p.118

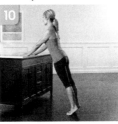

Standing Stretch

Triceps Foldover p.120

IT Band Stretch with a Twist p.121

Crescent Lunge with Chest Opener p.122

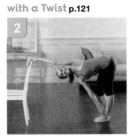

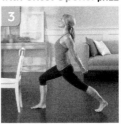

(continued)

Days 5 & 7 *(cont'd)*

Standing Stretch (cont'd)

Heel to Seat Stretch p.123

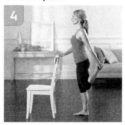

4

Figure 4 p.124

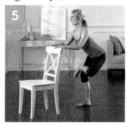

5

Mat Workout

Bridge Lifts p.162

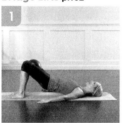

1

Bridge Lifts with Ball Hold p.164

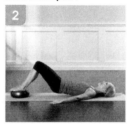

2

All Fours Levers Large p.166

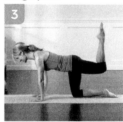

3

All Fours Levers 1 Inch p.168

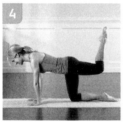

4

Upright Core Twists p.170

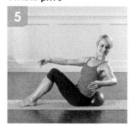

5

Core Rolls p.172

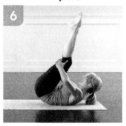

6

Incline Core Knee Marches p.174

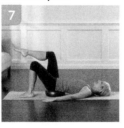

7

Incline Core Knee Catches p.176

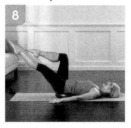

8

Bridge Lift Hold p.178

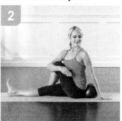

Seated Twist p.179

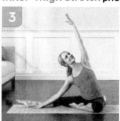

Side-Body and Inner-Thigh Stretch p.180

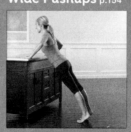

Staff Pose Deltoid Stretch p.181

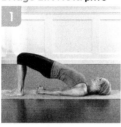

Modified Camel p.182

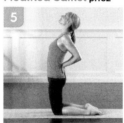

Crisscross Seated Neck Stretch p.183

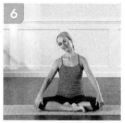

MOVE ALL DAY!

Choose among these barre3 Boosts and move for 1 minute every day this week:

Push-Pulls p.190

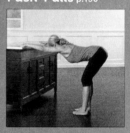

Horse Pose Pliés p.100

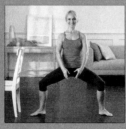

Wide Pushups p.154

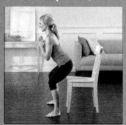

Sumo Squats p.116

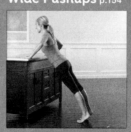

Raising the Barre

SARAH LA DU

AGE: 36   **POUNDS LOST:** 13   **INCHES LOST:** 9, *including 3¾ from her waist and 3 from her hips*

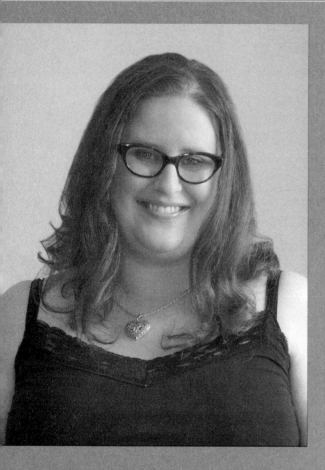

I was raised as a vegetarian who occasionally had fish. I've still never had a burger, steak, or fried chicken, and growing up I wasn't allowed white flour, refined sugar, or obviously processed food of any kind. Holidays like Easter or Halloween were candy free—I would eat banana chips instead. I never really developed a sweet tooth, but I love cheese. And croissants. And pasta. And cocktails. I started to gain weight at around age 23 and never stopped. A couple of complicated medical conditions only accelerated this and made me feel hopeless. My doctor actually told me it didn't matter what I did, that I would never lose weight. So I gave up and gradually watched the scale climb to 237 pounds.

Recently, I decided to give weight loss one last try. Because of my eating history, the Love Your Lower Body program resonated with me. It was also one of the first "diet" programs I've ever seen that seemed doable without eating meat. But my biggest surprise was that I started to want to work out. After 8 weeks on this plan, there are certain times of day where my body needs to move and get in some exercise. I've never felt that way before. Historically, I hate exercise. So wanting and needing to work out daily was a huge surprise. During the 8 weeks, I worked out 6 days a week, every week, exactly as prescribed. By the second month, it was harder to *not* work out on my rest day than it was *to* work out on the other days of the week.

My favorite part of the plan is definitely the flexibility. I love that there are so many ways to make a DIY bowl and that if there's a salad recipe that calls for chicken, I can substitute chickpeas. The workouts are doable regardless of fitness level. There's a modification—or five—for pretty much everything. When things got challenging, I learned to give myself some space, take a few breaths, and come back stronger for the finish. I didn't force myself to do what was too hard, but I didn't stop and give up either, which was life changing.

I started out barely able to do 10 minutes at a time. Now I can make it through 60 minutes straight. I gave up cheese for a month, and I've swapped Greek yogurt for sour cream. I'm no longer exhausted after work, and I feel stronger now and a lot less hopeless. I used to think I got the short genetic straw and there was nothing I could do about it. This is the first time in a really long time that I've felt real hope and had the faith in myself that I could do it.

I LOVE MY LOWER BODY *because*:

My calves have gone from a slope, to a shelf, to what actually looks like the outline of the muscle. I've never had that before, even when I was super-thin and active. I also love my waist and core. Not so much the look of it, but I love that the strength there has taken a lot of strain off my lower back. As my core has gotten stronger, so has my lower back. I also love that my stomach muscles tend to engage all throughout the day without me thinking about it. Whenever I start to slouch or I've been sitting too long, I can feel those muscles engage, and as a result, I automatically feel a bit stronger, sit a bit taller, and have better posture. All because my stomach doesn't like being lazy anymore.

Chapter 7

The LOVE Your LOWER BODY Recipes

EAT GOOD, FEEL GOOD. THAT'S THE PREMISE BEHIND THE 50 RECIPES you'll find on the coming pages. A team of nutritionists and chefs helped me create meals and snacks that strike the perfect balance between delicious and nutritious. Some are variations of tried-and-true favorites like Chicken Tacos and chopped salad; others might feel a bit more exotic, such as the Tropical Quinoa Detox Smoothie or the Tzatziki Chicken with Greek Salad. By working with a range of whole foods, we have options to fit every taste, preference, and eating restriction.

I encourage you to try new recipes and repeat favorites as you find them. To cut down on your time in the kitchen, I've made many recipes that can be paired. You might make Pork Lettuce Cups one evening, then use the leftover meat in the Pork Rice Bowl for the next day's lunch. (I'm a big fan of these "bowls" for lunch. Just take your protein from dinner and add it to a mix of grains and greens.) Making larger batches to freeze or eat multiple days in a row can help you become more efficient around mealtimes. On days that you simply don't have time to cook, turn to my list of grab-and-go meals and snacks on page 53 for healthy time-saving options.

Do It Yourself

When I have a bunch of produce to use up or a few picky eaters to feed, I make mealtimes a DIY experience. This works great for smoothies, muesli, omelets, salads, bowls, pizza, and more. Lay out ingredients as you'd find them at a salad bar, then let each person craft his or her own dinner.

This chapter includes a few DIY recipes—formulas from which you can pick and choose your ingredients and that steer you toward getting a healthy balance of protein, fat, and fiber. These are just jumping-off points—feel free to get creative!

Smoothies

Breakfast

Lunch

Dinner

Snacks

DiY Smoothie

Prep Time: 5 minutes • Total Time: 7 minutes • Makes 2 servings

Start with your base:

- 1 cup water, coconut milk, nut milk, or coconut water
- 1 cup ice

Add your greens:

- 1 cup spinach, kale, braising greens, celery, parsley, or cilantro

Add your fruit:

- 1 cup blackberries, blueberries, boysenberries, raspberries, or strawberries
- 1 cup apple, cherries, kiwifruit, mango chunks, peaches, pear, or pineapple

Add 1 to 3 of these proteins and healthy fats:

- ¼ cup seeds, nuts, or nut butter (such as almonds, Brazil nuts, sunflower seeds, or walnuts)
- 2 tablespoons chia seeds
- 2 tablespoons hemp seeds
- 2 tablespoons ground flaxseed

Add 1 of these natural sweeteners (optional):

- ½ banana
- 4–6 pitted dates
- 2 tablespoons maple syrup

Add other flavors as desired:

- 1 teaspoon cinnamon
- 1 teaspoon vanilla extract
- 1 teaspoon fresh ginger
- 2 tablespoons freshly squeezed lemon juice

Sadie's Pick

Here's one of my favorite smoothie combinations.

For my base:
1 cup water
1 cup almond milk
1 cup ice

For my greens:
1 cup spinach

For my fruit:
1 cup frozen boysenberries

For my protein and healthy fat:
2 tablespoons ground flaxseed
2 tablespoons hemp seeds
¼ cup Brazil nuts

To sweeten and add flavor:
½ frozen banana
½ teaspoon cinnamon
½ teaspoon vanilla

Per serving: 586 calories, 40 g total fat, 6 g saturated fat, 45 g carbohydrates, 16 g dietary fiber, 18 g protein, 223 mg sodium

In a high-speed blender, process all chosen ingredients for 1 to 2 minutes, or until well blended.

SMOOTHIES

Tropical Quinoa Detox Smoothie

Prep Time: 5 minutes • Total Time: 7 minutes • **Makes 2 servings**

- ½ cup cooked quinoa
- ½ cup frozen spinach or kale (or 2 cups fresh)
- 1½ cups frozen pineapple chunks
- 1 banana
- 1 cup coconut milk
- 1 tablespoon lime juice
- 1 tablespoon cilantro leaves
- ⅓ cup cucumber
- ¼ cup whole milk plain yogurt
- 2–4 pitted dates (optional)
- 2 tablespoons chia seeds, ground
- 2 cups ice cubes

In a high-speed blender, process all the ingredients for 1 to 2 minutes, or until well blended.

Per serving: 575 calories, 30 g total fat, 23 g saturated fat, 76 g carbohydrates, 11 g dietary fiber, 10 g protein, 79 mg sodium

Pumpkin Spice Smoothie

Prep Time: 5 minutes • Total Time: 7 minutes • Makes 2 servings

- 1 ripe frozen banana
- ½ cup almond milk
- ½ cup coconut milk
- ½ cup pumpkin puree
- ¼ cup almond butter
- 2 teaspoons pure maple syrup
- ¾ teaspoon cinnamon
- ⅛ teaspoon nutmeg
- 1 cup ice cubes

In a high-speed blender, process all the ingredients for 1 to 2 minutes, or until well blended.

Per serving: 412 calories, 30 g total fat, 13 g saturated fat, 33 g carbohydrates, 8 g dietary fiber, 9 g protein, 121 mg sodium

Almond Date Cinnamon Smoothie

Prep Time: 5 minutes • Total Time: 7 minutes • Makes 2 servings

- **1 ripe frozen banana**
- **5 pitted dates**
- **¼ cup almond butter**
- **1 teaspoon cinnamon**
- **1 cup coconut milk**
- **½ cup almond milk**
- **½ cup water**
- **1 cup ice cubes**

In a high-speed blender, process all the ingredients for 1 to 2 minutes, or until well blended.

Per serving: 651 calories, 42 g total fat, 24 g saturated fat, 71 g carbohydrates, 11 g dietary fiber, 11 g protein, 128 mg sodium

Eggs with Sautéed Spinach and Mushrooms

Prep Time: 10 minutes • Total Time: 25 minutes • **Makes 2 servings**

2½ tablespoons olive oil, divided

4 eggs

4 cloves garlic, diced

2 cups mushrooms, diced

8 cups spinach, rinsed and patted dry

¼ teaspoon salt

⅛ teaspoon ground black pepper

Avocado slices for garnish

Cherry tomatoes for garnish

1. Heat 2 tablespoons of the oil in a skillet over medium heat.
2. Scramble the eggs with a fork in a bowl. Pour the eggs into the skillet and cook until no longer runny, flipping once. Remove the eggs before they begin to brown and set aside.
3. Heat the remaining ½ tablespoon oil in the skillet. Add the garlic and cook for 2 minutes. Add the mushrooms and cook for 3 to 5 minutes until softened, stirring occasionally. Add the spinach, salt, and pepper and cook for about 4 minutes until the spinach is wilted, stirring frequently.
4. Scramble the eggs into the spinach mixture and cook over medium heat until the eggs are firm. Garnish with the avocado and tomatoes.

Per serving: 347 calories, 28 g total fat, 6 g saturated fat, 10 g carbohydrates, 4 g dietary fiber, 19 g protein, 528 mg sodium

BREAKFAST

Skinny Omelet with Greens

Prep Time: 5 minutes • Total Time: 10 minutes • **Makes 2 servings**

> 4 **eggs**
> 2 **pinches of sea salt**
> 2 **teaspoons olive oil**
> 1¾ **cups (about 1 large handful) arugula or spinach, chopped**
> ¼ **cup basil leaves**
> 2 **teaspoons balsamic vinegar**
> **Ground black pepper**

1. In a small bowl, beat the eggs and salt.
2. Heat a medium nonstick skillet over medium heat. Brush lightly with the oil and pour in the egg mixture.
3. Swirl the pan so the eggs spread evenly in a very thin layer. Let set for 2 minutes. Run a spatula underneath the omelet and slide it out of the pan onto a lined baking sheet.
4. Place the arugula or spinach and basil on top of the omelet and roll it away from you. Cut it in half and warm slightly in the oven if you prefer the greens wilted. Season with a drizzle of the vinegar and add pepper to taste.

Per serving: 192 calories, 14 g total fat, 4 g saturated fat, 2 g carbohydrates, 0 g dietary fiber, 13 g protein, 245 mg sodium

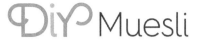 Muesli

Prep Time: 5 minutes • Total Time: 5 minutes • Makes 2 servings

Start with your base:

> 2 **cups old-fashioned rolled oats**
> **Pinch of cinnamon**
> **Pinch of nutmeg**

Pick 1 ingredient from each category:

> ½ **cup chopped nuts (almonds, hazelnuts, or walnuts)**
> 2 **tablespoons seeds (chia, ground flaxseed, pumpkin, or sunflower)**
> 2 **tablespoons dried fruit (blueberries, currants, goji berries, or raisins)**
> ½ **cup fresh berries (blackberries, blueberries, or raspberries)**

Choose 1 optional sweetener:

> ½ **cup finely shredded coconut flakes (also a good fat source)**
> 4 **chopped dates**
> 1 **tablespoon dark chocolate chips**

Combine the oats, cinnamon, and nutmeg with your choice of DIY ingredients. Serve with 1 cup whole milk yogurt, whole milk, coconut milk, or nut milk such as almond milk. Or, to serve warm, pour 1 cup boiling water over ingredients.

Sadie's Pick

Here's one of my favorite muesli combinations.

For my base:
2 cups old-fashioned rolled oats
Pinch of cinnamon
Pinch of nutmeg

For my additional ingredients (1 ingredient from each category):
½ cup chopped walnuts
2 tablespoons sunflower seeds
2 tablespoons dried goji berries
½ cup fresh blueberries (when in season)

I like this with almond milk.

Per serving: 575 calories, 22 g total fat, 1 g saturated fat, 73 g carbohydrates, 18 g dietary fiber, 23 g protein, 26 mg sodium

Sweet Rice Porridge

Prep Time: 5 minutes • Total Time: 10 minutes • Makes 2 servings

2 cups cooked brown rice or quinoa, warmed

1 cup almond milk

2 tablespoons chopped walnuts

2 tablespoons ground flaxseed

2 teaspoons maple syrup

2 teaspoons cinnamon

Pinch of nutmeg

½ cup fresh fruit such as blueberries or strawberries

1. In a medium saucepan over medium-low heat, combine the rice or quinoa, almond milk, walnuts, flaxseed, syrup, cinnamon, and nutmeg. Heat gently, stirring frequently, until hot. Alternatively, combine the ingredients in a microwaveable bowl, cover, and microwave on high power in 30-second increments. Stir after each increment until the porridge is hot.

2. Top with the fresh fruit.

TIP: This porridge is a great choice when you have leftover rice from the night before.

Per serving: 385 calories, 11 g total fat, 1 g saturated fat, 65 g carbohydrates, 9 g dietary fiber, 8 g protein, 81 mg sodium

Savory Rice Porridge

Prep Time: 5 minutes • Total Time: 10 minutes • **Makes 2 servings**

2 cups cooked brown rice or quinoa, warmed

1 cup fresh spinach

1 tablespoon butter, olive oil, or coconut butter

2 eggs

Dash of salt and pepper

1. Divide the warm rice or quinoa between 2 bowls and top each with ½ cup spinach.
2. In a medium skillet over medium heat, warm the butter, oil, or coconut butter. Add the eggs and cook over easy until the whites are opaque, then carefully turn without breaking the yolks. Cook for 10 more seconds.
3. Top each bowl's spinach with an over-easy egg and season with salt and pepper. The spinach will wilt under the egg.

Per serving: 346 calories, 12 g total fat, 6 g saturated fat, 48 g carbohydrates, 4 g dietary fiber, 11 g protein, 216 mg sodium

Quinoa Coconut Cereal

Prep Time: 5 minutes • Total Time: 25 minutes • **Makes 2 servings**

- 1 **cup water**
- ½ **cup quinoa, rinsed well and drained**
- 1½ **cups almond or coconut milk**
- 2 **tablespoons sesame seeds**
- 2 **tablespoons shredded coconut**
- 1 **tablespoon raw honey or maple syrup**
- ½ **teaspoon cinnamon**
- ½ **cup fruit of choice, such as mangoes or strawberries, sliced for serving**

1. In a medium saucepan, bring the water to a boil. Add the quinoa with a pinch of salt. Reduce the heat, cover, and simmer for 15 minutes, or until the water is absorbed and the quinoa is opened and soft. Turn off the heat and steam the quinoa for 3 minutes with the lid on.

2. Remove the lid and stir in the almond or coconut milk, seeds, coconut, honey or syrup, and cinnamon. Cook over medium heat for 2 minutes.

3. Taste and adjust for seasonings. Top with the fruit and enjoy!

Per serving: 333 calories, 11 g total fat, 3 g saturated fat, 53 g carbohydrates, 6 g dietary fiber, 9 g protein, 136 mg sodium

Buckwheat Buttermilk Pancakes with Blueberries

Prep Time: 5 minutes • Total Time: 25 minutes • **Makes 2 servings**

- 2 teaspoons butter
- ⅔ cup buckwheat flour
- ¼ cup brown rice flour
- ¼ cup tapioca flour
- 2 tablespoons ground flaxseed
- 1 teaspoon baking soda
- ¼ teaspoon sea salt
- 1⅓ cups organic buttermilk
- 2 tablespoons unsalted butter, melted
- 1 egg
- 1 teaspoon maple syrup, plus additional for topping
- ⅔ cup blueberries
- ¼ cup whole milk plain yogurt

1. In a cast-iron skillet over medium-low heat, melt the 2 teaspoons butter.
2. In a bowl, whisk together the flours, flaxseed, baking soda, and salt until thoroughly incorporated.
3. In a second, larger bowl, whip together the buttermilk, melted butter, the egg, and syrup.
4. Stir the dry ingredients into the buttermilk mixture. Fold in the blueberries.
5. Using a ladle or measuring cup, pour several 4" to 5" pancakes into the skillet. When they are bubbling around the edges, after 2 to 3 minutes, flip and cook for an additional 2 minutes, or until golden brown and thoroughly cooked. Serve with the yogurt and additional maple syrup.

TIP: This recipe also works well when the batter is refrigerated, covered, overnight.

Per serving (4 pancakes): 620 calories, 25 g total fat, 13 g saturated fat, 86 g carbohydrates, 8 g dietary fiber, 18 g protein, 1,060 mg sodium

Frittata Muffins

Prep Time: 5 minutes • Total Time: 25 minutes • Makes 2 servings

- **4 eggs**
- **1 tablespoon whole milk or canned coconut milk**
- **1 tablespoon olive oil**
- **¼ small red onion, finely chopped**
- **2 cups loosely packed spinach, arugula, or kale, chopped**
- **⅛ teaspoon sea salt**
- **⅛ teaspoon ground black pepper**

1. Preheat the oven to 350°F. Lightly oil 6 paper liners and place in a 6-cup muffin pan.
2. In a large bowl, beat the eggs and milk or coconut milk until evenly mixed.
3. In a small skillet over medium heat, warm the oil. Cook the onion; spinach, arugula, or kale; and the salt and pepper. Once the greens wilt, add them to the egg mixture, stirring to combine.
4. Pour into the muffin liners, filling about two-thirds full. Bake for 13 minutes, or until puffed and golden brown. Cool and enjoy for breakfast on the go.

Per serving (3 muffins): 216 calories, 17 g total fat, 4 g saturated fat, 3 g carbohydrates, 1 g dietary fiber, 13 g protein, 305 mg sodium

Spicy Harvest Soup

Prep Time: 10 minutes • Total Time: 35 minutes • **Makes 4 servings**

- 3 sprigs fresh thyme
- 2 sprigs fresh rosemary
- 1 sprig fresh sage
- 1 whole hot pepper (Scotch bonnet or habanero chile, very hot; red chile, less hot; or yellow chile, mild)
- 1 teaspoon olive oil
- 1 small sweet onion, diced
- 2 cloves garlic, diced
- 4 cups low-sodium chicken or vegetable broth
- 1 small butternut squash (about 1 pound), peeled, seeded, and chopped into 1" cubes
- ½ head cauliflower, chopped
- 1 zucchini, chopped
- 1 can (15 ounces) navy or great Northern beans, rinsed and drained
- ½ teaspoon sea salt
- ½ teaspoon ground black pepper
- 1 avocado, cubed
- Sour cream or whole milk plain yogurt (optional)

1. In a square of cheesecloth, lay the thyme, rosemary, sage, and chile pepper. Tie into a bundle or secure with kitchen string. Set aside.
2. In a large soup pot over medium heat, heat the oil. Add the onion and garlic and cook until golden, about 8 minutes. Add the broth, squash, and herb bundle. Bring to a boil. Reduce the heat and simmer until the squash begins to get tender, about 10 minutes. Add the cauliflower, zucchini, and beans and simmer 10 minutes until the vegetables are very tender.
3. Remove the herb bundle. Puree the soup with a handheld immersion blender (or in a large blender, in batches, if necessary). Season with the salt and pepper. Serve topped with the avocado and a dollop of the sour cream or yogurt, if using.

Per serving: 247 calories, 7 g total fat, 1 g saturated fat, 39 g carbohydrates, 10 g dietary fiber, 11 g protein, 620 mg sodium

LUNCH

Chicken and Kale Soup

Prep Time: 10 minutes • Total Time: 50 minutes • **Makes 6 servings**

- 1 tablespoon olive oil, divided
- 1 pound ground chicken
- 1 large onion, chopped
- 4 cloves garlic, chopped
- 5 cups chicken broth
- 1 head cauliflower, cored and chopped into small pieces
- 1 large bunch kale, leaves removed from spine and chopped into small to medium-size pieces
- ½ teaspoon sea salt
- ¼ teaspoon ground black pepper

1. Add ½ tablespoon of the oil to a large Dutch oven or soup pot and heat over medium heat. Add the chicken and cook until browned and cooked through, about 8 minutes. Remove from the pot and set aside.

2. Add the remaining ½ tablespoon oil to the pot and heat, loosening up browned bits from the bottom with a spoon or spatula. Add the onion and garlic and cook for 4 minutes, or until the onion softens and becomes translucent and the garlic browns.

3. Add the broth and bring to a boil. Reduce the heat. Add the cauliflower and simmer for 25 minutes, or until the cauliflower is tender. Add the kale and simmer for 4 minutes, or until the kale is tender.

4. Season with the salt and pepper. Serve immediately or refrigerate in smaller containers to enjoy later.

Per serving: 193 calories, 10 g total fat, 2 g saturated fat, 12 g carbohydrates, 3 g dietary fiber, 18 g protein, 937 mg sodium

$\mathcal{D}i\mathcal{P}$ Salad and Dressing

Prep Time: 10 minutes • Total Time: 20 minutes • **Makes 4 servings**

DIY Salad

8 cups of at least 3 lettuces or greens: arugula, Belgian endive, butter lettuce, cabbage (green Napa, red, savoy), curly endive, dandelion, mesclun, mizuna, mustard greens, radicchio, red leaf lettuce, romaine, spinach, or watercress

4 cups of at least 4 veggies, herbs, or seeds: avocado, beets (steamed, roasted, or grated raw), broccoli (raw or gently steamed), carrots, celery, cucumber, fennel bulb (chopped or sliced), herbs (chives, cilantro, dill, mint, oregano, or parsley), radishes, seeds (pumpkin, raw sunflower, or sesame), snap peas, spring onions, or sprouts

2 cups of 1 protein source: chicken, fish, hard-cooked eggs, legumes, nuts, or seeds

DIY Dressing

½ cup chopped fresh herbs (basil, chives, cilantro, dill, or parsley)

¼ cup vinegar (apple cider, balsamic, or red wine)

1 cup olive oil

½ teaspoon sea salt

½ teaspoon ground black pepper (optional)

1–2 cloves garlic, chopped (optional)

1–2 teaspoons Dijon mustard (optional)

Sadie's Pick

Here's my favorite salad.

For my base:
8 cups arugula, butter lettuce, and red leaf lettuce
1 avocado
1 cup roasted beets
¼ cup sunflower seeds
1½ cups diced grilled chicken

For my dressing:
¼ cup chopped fresh parsley
¼ cup chopped fresh basil
¼ cup balsamic vinegar
1 cup olive oil
½ teaspoon sea salt
½ teaspoon ground black pepper
1 clove garlic, chopped
1 teaspoon Dijon mustard

Per serving: 599 calories, 54 g total fat, 8 g saturated fat, 13 g carbohydrates, 5 g dietary fiber, 21 g protein, 333 mg sodium

1. **TO MAKE THE SALAD:** In a large bowl, combine your choice of lettuces or greens. Top with the veggies, herbs, or seeds and protein.
2. **TO MAKE THE DRESSING:** Combine your choice of ingredients in a blender or food processor and pulse until mixed. Pour all but ¼ to ⅓ cup over the salad and toss.
3. Save the remaining dressing sealed in a jar in the refrigerator for up to 1 week.

MAKE IT YOUR OWN: GO MEATLESS

Many of the Love Your Lower Body recipes fit into vegan and vegetarian eating plans, but even the ones that contain animal products can be easily altered to suit your palate. Here are our recommended substitutions for popular ingredients.

- Eggs in baked goods: Substitute ¼ cup applesauce for 1 egg.

- Meat or eggs as a main protein source: Beans and legumes are good stand-ins; tofu and tempeh can be used in moderation.

- Milk: Try rice milk, coconut milk, almond milk, oat milk, or soy milk instead.

- Cheese: Get a similar flavor from tofu cheese, rice cheese, almond cheese, or nutritional yeast.

- Yogurt or sour cream: Satisfy your craving with soy yogurt.

Polenta Salad

Prep Time: 5 minutes • Total Time: 30 minutes • **Makes 2 servings**

- **1** small yellow or green zucchini, cut into ¼" slices
- **2** cups mushrooms, sliced
- **1** red bell pepper, seeded and cut into chunks
- **1** cup grape tomatoes
- **1** tablespoon olive oil
- **⅛** teaspoon ground black pepper
- **¼** teaspoon sea salt, divided
- **1** tablespoon balsamic vinegar
- **1** cup coarse polenta (corn grits), cooked
- **¼** cup hummus

1. Preheat the oven to 450°F. Mist a large rimmed baking sheet with nonstick cooking spray.
2. Place the zucchini, mushrooms, bell pepper, and tomatoes on the baking sheet. Drizzle with the oil and sprinkle with the black pepper and ⅛ teaspoon of the salt. Toss to combine. Arrange the vegetables in a single layer and roast for 20 minutes, turning once, or until the vegetables are golden and softened and the tomatoes release their juices.
3. Toss with the remaining ⅛ teaspoon salt and the vinegar.
4. Divide the cooked polenta between 2 bowls. Top with the roasted vegetables and hummus.

TIP: Use leftover polenta from last night's dinner if you cooked Lemon-Garlic Chicken and Polenta with Roasted Vegetables (page 268).

Per serving: 331 calories, 12 g total fat, 2 g saturated fat, 49 g carbohydrates, 7 g dietary fiber, 10 g protein, 852 mg sodium

Mediterranean Quinoa Salad with Carrot Fries

Prep Time: 5 minutes • Total Time: 30 minutes • **Makes 2 servings**

Carrot Fries

- 3 medium to large carrots, quartered lengthwise, then cut crosswise into 2½"–3" sticks
- 1 tablespoon olive oil
- ¼ teaspoon sea salt

Salad

- 1 cup water
- ½ cup dry quinoa, rinsed well and drained
- 1 can (15 ounces) chickpeas, rinsed and drained
- 3 scallions, thinly sliced
- 1 cup Italian parsley, finely chopped
- ⅓ cup fresh mint, finely chopped
- 1 cucumber, seeded and finely chopped
- 1 cup baby spinach
- ¼ cup olive oil
- ¼ cup lemon juice
- ¼ teaspoon sea salt (more to taste)

1. **TO MAKE THE CARROT FRIES:** Preheat the oven to 425°F. Coat a baking sheet with nonstick cooking spray.

2. In a medium bowl, toss the carrots, oil, and salt together. Spread on the baking sheet. Bake for 12 to 15 minutes until golden brown, turning once. Remove from the oven and set aside.

3. **TO MAKE THE SALAD:** In a saucepan, bring the water and quinoa to a boil, uncovered. Reduce the heat, cover, and simmer for 15 minutes. Turn off the heat and steam the quinoa for 5 minutes. Remove the lid and fluff with a fork.

4. In a large bowl, combine the cooked quinoa, chickpeas, scallions, parsley, mint, cucumber, spinach, oil, lemon juice, and salt. Enjoy immediately or keep in the fridge—great chilled for an easy salad. Serve with the carrot fries.

Per serving: 687 calories, 43 g total fat, 6 g saturated fat, 66 g carbohydrates, 16 g dietary fiber, 17 g protein, 894 mg sodium

Black Bean Bowls with Cumin-Lime Dressing

Prep Time: 15 minutes • Total Time: 30 minutes • **Makes 4 servings**

2 cups water

1 cup quinoa, rinsed well and drained

¼ cup freshly squeezed lime juice

⅓ cup extra-virgin olive oil

1 large clove garlic, minced

½ teaspoon ground cumin

2 teaspoons honey

⅛ teaspoon crushed red-pepper flakes

1 can (14.5 ounces) black beans, rinsed and drained

1 avocado, diced

1 small red onion, finely chopped

½ head purple cabbage, shredded

½ cup cilantro, chopped

1. In a medium saucepan, combine the water and quinoa. Bring to a boil. Reduce the heat, cover, and simmer for 15 minutes, or until the water has absorbed and the quinoa is light and fluffy.

2. Meanwhile, prepare the Cumin-Lime Dressing. In a small bowl, or in a jar with a lid, combine the lime juice, oil, garlic, cumin, honey, and pepper flakes. Whisk together or shake until well mixed.

3. Transfer the quinoa to a serving bowl. Combine with the black beans, avocado, onion, and cabbage. Gently stir in the dressing and cilantro. Enjoy warm, at room temperature, or cold.

Per serving: 484 calories, 27 g total fat, 4 g saturated fat, 55 g carbohydrates, 11 g dietary fiber, 12 g protein, 117 mg sodium

Tuna Niçoise Salad with Dijon Vinaigrette

Prep Time: 10 minutes • Total Time: 20 minutes • **Makes 2 servings**

Dressing

- 3 tablespoons lemon juice
- 1 tablespoon Dijon mustard
- 1 tablespoon honey
- ¼ cup olive oil
- ¼ teaspoon sea salt
- ¼ teaspoon ground black pepper

Salad

- 1 tablespoon olive oil
- 1 tuna steak (8 ounces), halved
- 1 cup green beans, strings removed, halved
- 1 head romaine lettuce, torn into bite-size pieces
- 2 Roma tomatoes, quartered
- 2 hard-cooked eggs, quartered
- 1 small red onion, sliced very thin
- ¼ cup Niçoise olives

1. **TO MAKE THE DRESSING:** In a small bowl, whisk together the lemon juice, mustard, honey, oil, salt, and pepper.

2. **TO MAKE THE SALAD:** Heat a large skillet over medium-high heat, add the oil, and sear the tuna for 2 to 3 minutes on each side, or until just opaque. Remove from the skillet. When cool enough to handle, slice the tuna into ¼"- to ½"-thick slices.

3. Place a steamer basket in a large pot with 1" water. Bring to a boil over high heat. Steam the beans in the basket until fork-tender, about 5 minutes, then run under cold water to cool.

4. Arrange the lettuce in 2 bowls. Place little piles of the beans, tomatoes, eggs, onion, and olives on the salad greens. Top with the seared tuna and drizzle with the dressing.

Per serving: 699 calories, 50 g total fat, 7 g saturated fat, 33 g carbohydrates, 8 g dietary fiber, 37 g protein, 934 mg sodium

Grilled Fish Salad

Prep Time: 5 minutes • Total Time: 5 minutes • Makes 2 servings

- 5 ounces grilled white fish, such as tilapia, cut into bite-size chunks
- 2 cups premixed cabbage slaw
- 1 cup baby spinach
- ¼ cup hummus
- 2 tablespoons sunflower seeds

In a large bowl, gently combine the fish, slaw, and spinach. Divide between 2 bowls. Top each with half of the hummus and 1 tablespoon sunflower seeds.

TIP: Use leftover grilled fish and slaw from last night's dinner if you cooked Grilled Fish Tacos with Slaw (page 260).

Per serving: 213 calories, 9 g total fat, 1 g saturated fat, 11 g carbohydrates, 4 g dietary fiber, 22 g protein, 236 mg sodium

Zesty Chicken Salad

Prep Time: 5 minutes • Total Time: 10 minutes • **Makes 4 servings**

- 2 cups diced cooked chicken breast
- 1 cup diced dill pickles
- 1 tablespoon finely diced onion
- ¼ cup cilantro
- ½ tablespoon Dijon mustard
- 2 tablespoons whole milk plain yogurt
- ½ teaspoon paprika
- ¼ cup dried cranberries or raisins
- ½ apple, chopped
- ⅛ teaspoon sea salt
- 4 cups mixed greens

1. In a medium-size bowl, mix together the chicken, pickles, onion, cilantro, mustard, yogurt, paprika, cranberries or raisins, apple, and salt.
2. Place 1 cup of greens on each plate and top with equal portions of the chicken salad mixture.

TIP: Make this dish with leftover chicken from last night's dinner if you cooked Brined Chicken Breast with Roasted Broccoli (page 270). Or, for a vegetarian version, use tempeh.

Per serving: 175 calories, 3 g total fat, 1 g saturated fat, 13 g carbohydrates, 3 g dietary fiber, 24 g protein, 506 mg sodium

Rough-Chopped Salad with Chicken and Pistachio-Herb Vinaigrette

Prep Time: 15 minutes • Total Time: 45 minutes • **Makes 4 servings**

- 2 boneless, skinless chicken breasts (6 ounces each)
- 2 tablespoons + ¼ cup olive oil
- 1 teaspoon sea salt, divided
- ½ teaspoon ground black pepper, divided
- 1 cup shelled unsalted pistachios
- 1 red onion, sliced
- 1 tablespoon chopped fresh sage
- 1 tablespoon chopped fresh rosemary
- 3 cloves garlic, minced
- ¼ cup red wine vinegar
- 4 ounces (4 cups) red leaf lettuce (or any mix of fresh, dark salad greens, such as kale)
- 2 ounces (2 cups) spinach
- 1 yellow squash, chopped into bite-size pieces
- 10 radishes, thinly sliced
- 2 carrots, chopped into bite-size pieces
- 2 avocados, chopped into bite-size pieces
- 2 tomatoes, chopped into bite-size pieces
- 1 orange, cut into 4 wedges

1. Coat a grill rack or broiler-pan rack with cooking spray. Preheat the grill or broiler. Lightly coat the chicken with 1 tablespoon of the oil and season with ½ teaspoon of the salt and ¼ teaspoon of the pepper. Place the rack 6" from the heat source. Cook the chicken, turning once, for 8 minutes, or until a thermometer inserted in the thickest portion registers 165°F and the juices run clear. Set aside.

2. In a medium skillet over medium heat, lightly toast the pistachios until fragrant, about 5 minutes. Set aside in a medium bowl.

3. Return the skillet to medium heat and add 1 tablespoon oil. Cook the onion, stirring occasionally, until golden, about 10 minutes. Add the sage, rosemary, and garlic. Gently stir until the warmed herbs release a bit of aroma. Remove from the heat and add the herb mixture to the reserved pistachios.

4. In a small bowl, combine the vinegar and the remaining $1/4$ cup oil. Add to the onion mixture. Season with the remaining salt and pepper. Let this dressing stand so the flavors combine while you prep the rest of the dish.

5. Wash, dry, and shred the lettuce and spinach into short 1"-wide strips. Place in a large bowl. Add the squash, radishes, carrots, avocados, and tomatoes and gently toss with the greens.

6. Divide the salad mixture among 4 plates. Squeeze 1 orange wedge over each serving. Shred the chicken and place equal portions across the top of each plate. Pour the dressing over each serving.

TIP: Substitute chickpeas or white beans for a vegetarian option, or omit the chicken and serve alongside a serving of fish or other protein.

Per serving: 639 calories, 48 g total fat, 7 g saturated fat, 30 g carbohydrates, 12 g dietary fiber, 29 g protein, 564 mg sodium

Sirloin Steak Salad with Avocado

Prep Time: **10 minutes** • Total Time: **20 minutes** • **Makes 2 servings**

½ **pound sirloin steak**

½ **teaspoon sea salt, divided**

½ **teaspoon ground black pepper, divided**

2 **tablespoons coconut oil or safflower oil, divided**

1 **red bell pepper, diced**

1 **avocado, diced**

1 **rib celery, diced**

2 **scallions, chopped**

2 **ounces (2 cups) baby spinach**

1 **tablespoon lemon or lime juice**

1. Season the steak with ¼ teaspoon each of the salt and black pepper.

2. Heat a medium skillet over medium-high heat. When hot, add 1 tablespoon of the coconut or safflower oil. Add the bell pepper and cook for 2 minutes, then remove and set aside in a medium bowl.

3. To the same skillet, add the remaining oil and the seasoned steak. Cook for 3 minutes per side (for medium-rare), or until a thermometer inserted in the center registers 145°F for medium-rare/160°F for medium/165°F for well-done. Let stand for 5 minutes before slicing.

4. Meanwhile, in a medium bowl, combine the cooked bell pepper with the avocado, celery, scallions, spinach, and lemon or lime juice. Season with the remaining salt and black pepper. You may add the oil liquid from the skillet to the salad for additional flavor.

5. Slice the steak on the diagonal and serve over the avocado-spinach salad.

Per serving: 423 calories, 30 g total fat, 15 g saturated fat, 15 g carbohydrates, 8 g dietary fiber, 28 g protein, 523 mg sodium

Pork Rice Bowls

Prep Time: 5 minutes • Total Time: 15 minutes • **Makes 2 servings**

- ¾ cups cooked brown rice
- ¼ cup (3 ounces) cooked and sliced pork
- 1 tablespoon tamari
- 1 tablespoon rice vinegar
- 1 teaspoon toasted sesame seeds
- 1 tablespoon toasted almond slices
- ½ avocado, chopped

  Any veggies in your refrigerator (leafy greens, carrots, cabbage, cucumber, onions, etc.), chopped

In a medium bowl, combine the rice, pork, tamari, vinegar, seeds, almonds, avocado, and chopped veggies. Toss and enjoy.

TIP: Use leftover pork from last night's dinner if you cooked Pork Lettuce Cups (page 275).

Per serving: 268 calories, 14 g total fat, 3 g saturated fat, 21 g carbohydrates, 4 g dietary fiber, 15 g protein, 497 mg sodium

Smoked Salmon Frittata

Prep Time: 5 minutes • Total Time: 30 minutes • **Makes 2 servings**

  4 eggs
  ¼ cup canned coconut milk
  3 teaspoons olive oil, divided
  ¼ small red onion, finely chopped
  ⅛ teaspoon sea salt
  ⅛ teaspoon ground black pepper
  4 ounces smoked salmon, flaked into pieces
  4 scallions, thinly sliced
  4 cups mixed greens
  1 teaspoon balsamic vinegar

1. Preheat the oven to 350°F.
2. In a medium bowl, beat the eggs and coconut milk until evenly mixed.
3. In a 7" cast-iron skillet over medium heat, warm 2 teaspoons of the oil. Add the onion, salt, and pepper and cook for 3 minutes. Remove the skillet from the heat. Stir the cooked onions, salmon, and scallions into the egg mixture until well combined.
4. Pour the mixture back into the skillet and bake for 15 minutes, or until puffed and golden brown. Cool and slice. Serve with a side of mixed greens tossed with the remaining 1 teaspoon oil and the vinegar.

Per serving: 493 calories, 29 g total fat, 11 g saturated fat, 9 g carbohydrates, 4 g dietary fiber, 50 g protein, 354 mg sodium

Chicken Tacos

Prep Time: 5 minutes • Total Time: 40 minutes • **Makes 4 servings**

- 2 teaspoons olive oil, divided
- 1 pound ground chicken
- 1 small onion, diced (about ½ cup)
- 2 cloves garlic, diced
- 1 teaspoon oregano
- 1 teaspoon cumin
- ½ teaspoon chili powder
- ½ teaspoon sea salt
- 1 can (15 ounces) pinto beans, black beans, or kidney beans, rinsed and drained
- 8 corn tortillas
- 1 cup cilantro, chopped
- ½ cup salsa of choice
- 1 avocado, sliced
- ¼ cup feta cheese (optional)

1. Heat 1 teaspoon of the olive oil in a skillet over medium heat. Add the chicken and cook, stirring occasionally, for about 8 minutes, or until no longer pink. Remove the chicken to a plate or bowl.

2. To the skillet, add the remaining oil. Add the onion and cook for 4 minutes, or until softened. Add the garlic and cook for 2 minutes. Add the oregano, cumin, chili powder, and salt and stir. Return the chicken to the skillet and combine with the onion mixture.

3. Add the beans to the skillet and heat through.

4. In a separate skillet, heat each tortilla for 3 minutes, flipping after 2 minutes, until puffed up and beginning to crisp. If the pan is large enough, heat 2 tortillas at a time.

5. Fill each tortilla with a small amount of the chicken mixture. Top each with 2 tablespoons of the cilantro, 1 tablespoon of the salsa, avocado slices, and ½ tablespoon of the cheese, if using.

Per serving (2 tacos): 450 calories, 21 g total fat, 6 g saturated fat, 41 g carbohydrates, 10 g dietary fiber, 29 g protein, 907 mg sodium

Southwest Chicken Collard Wrap

Prep Time: 10 minutes • Total Time: 40 minutes • **Makes 2 servings**

2 boneless, skinless chicken breasts (6–8 ounces each)

¼ teaspoon sea salt

¼ teaspoon ground black pepper

¼ teaspoon ground red pepper

1 tablespoon lime juice

4 large collard green leaves

1 teaspoon balsamic vinegar or lemon juice

1 carrot, shredded

½ cucumber, thinly sliced

¼ cup cilantro, chopped

1 avocado, sliced

½ cup salsa (optional)

Dash of hot sauce (optional)

1. Poach or roast the chicken, as desired. To poach, place the chicken in a medium saucepan and add enough water to cover. Salt the water, if desired. Bring to a boil, uncovered, and immediately reduce the heat. Simmer for 15 minutes, then remove the pan from the heat and allow to cool for 15 minutes. Remove the chicken to a cutting board. To roast, preheat the oven to 350°F. Place the chicken on a baking sheet and season with the salt, black pepper, red pepper, and lime juice. Bake for 25 minutes, or until a thermometer inserted in the thickest portion registers 165°F and the juices run clear.

2. Let the chicken rest while you prepare the wrap ingredients. When cool enough to handle, shred the breasts with two forks. (If the breasts were poached, season them with the salt, black pepper, red pepper, and lime juice.)

3. Meanwhile, soak the collard leaves in water with the vinegar or lemon juice for 10 minutes. Pat dry. Place one leaf on a cutting board, with the fatter part of the stem facing up. Remove the white part of the stem (the part without any leaf). With a paring knife, carefully "shave" the thickest part of the stem so that it's about as thick as the rest of the leaf. Repeat with remaining leaves.

4. Lay 2 leaves on a cutting board, spine side down, with the stem ends facing in opposite directions. Overlap them slightly so that they form one large leaf. Place half of the carrot, cucumber, cilantro, and avocado along the lower third of the leaves. Top with half of the shredded chicken.

5. Fold up the lower end of the collard leaf over the ingredients, tuck the sides in, and roll the leaf away from you. Secure with a toothpick, if necessary, and cut in half. Repeat with the remaining ingredients. Serve with the salsa or hot sauce, if using.

Per serving: 351 calories, 16 g total fat, 3 g saturated fat, 14 g carbohydrates, 9 g dietary fiber, 40 g protein, 434 mg sodium

Turkey-Avocado Lettuce Wrap

Prep Time: 10 minutes • Total Time: 10 minutes • **Makes 2 servings**

1 tablespoon finely chopped red onion

1½ teaspoons freshly squeezed lime juice

1½ teaspoons red wine vinegar

3 tablespoons freshly squeezed orange juice

Pinch of sea salt

Pinch of ground white pepper

4 teaspoons olive oil

1 ripe avocado, cut into ½" cubes

4 romaine or butter lettuce leaves, washed and patted dried

½ pound oven-roasted turkey, sliced and cut into strips

1. In a medium bowl, combine the onion, lime juice, vinegar, orange juice, salt, and pepper. Whisk in the oil.

2. Stir in the avocado cubes, being careful not to smash them.

3. To assemble the wraps, lay the lettuce leaves flat and layer with half of the turkey and half of the avocado salad. Wrap as you would a burrito.

Per serving: 375 calories, 21 g total fat, 3g saturated fat, 12 g carbohydrates, 7 g dietary fiber, 37 g protein, 121 mg sodium

Black Bean Chili

Prep Time: 10 minutes + soaking time for beans
• Total Time: 2 hours 30 minutes • **Makes 4 servings**

  1 pound dried black beans

  2 onions, chopped

  3 carrots, grated

  1 tablespoon olive oil

  6 cloves garlic, minced

  3 tablespoons chili powder

  1 tablespoon cumin

½–1 teaspoon red-pepper flakes

  1½ teaspoons oregano

  ¾ teaspoon cinnamon

  6 cups low-sodium organic chicken or veggie broth

½–1 cup water (based on how thick you like your chili)

  1 teaspoon sea salt

Toppings

  1 avocado, diced

  3 scallions, sliced thin

  ½ cup fresh cilantro, chopped

  1 tomato, diced

1. Soak the beans overnight in enough water to cover. Rinse, drain, and remove any pebbles.

2. In a large pot over medium heat, brown the onions and carrots in the oil for about 10 minutes. Add the garlic, chili powder, cumin, pepper flakes, oregano, and cinnamon. Cook, stirring, for 2 minutes.

3. Add the broth, beans, ½ cup water, and salt and bring to a boil. Reduce the heat and simmer partially covered for 2 hours, or until the beans are tender. Add more water if the consistency is too thick. Mash with a potato masher until lumpy.

4. Serve the bowls of chili topped with the avocado, scallions, cilantro, and tomato.

Per serving: 567 calories, 11 g total fat, 2 g saturated fat, 92 g carbohydrates, 30 g dietary fiber, 30 g protein, 546 mg sodium

Butternut Squash and Black Bean Bowl

Prep Time: 10 minutes • Total Time: 45 minutes • **Makes 4 servings**

1 butternut squash (3 pounds), peeled, seeded, and cut into ¾" cubes

2 tablespoons olive oil, divided

⅛ teaspoon sea salt

⅛ teaspoon ground black pepper

½ cup brown rice, uncooked

1 medium-size yellow onion, finely chopped

2 cloves garlic, minced

1 red bell pepper, seeded and chopped

2 teaspoons ground cumin

½–1 teaspoon ground red pepper

1 large tomato, diced

4 cups spinach

1 can (15 ounces) black beans, rinsed and drained

1. Preheat the oven to 425°F. Combine the squash, 1 tablespoon of the oil, the salt, and black pepper. Place on a baking sheet and roast in the oven for 20 minutes, turning halfway through the cooking time, or until the squash is fork-tender.

2. Meanwhile, cook the rice according to package directions.

3. In a large skillet over medium heat, heat the remaining oil. Add the onion and cook for about 5 minutes, or until golden brown and softened. Add the garlic, bell pepper, cumin, and red pepper. Cook for 2 minutes. Add the tomato, spinach, beans, and cooked squash to the pan. Stir until well combined.

4. Scoop ¼ cup rice into each of 4 bowls and top with the squash mixture.

Per serving: 374 calories, 9 g total fat, 1 g saturated fat, 70 g carbohydrates, 13 g dietary fiber, 10 g protein, 308 mg sodium

Veggie Tacos with Coriander-Orange Dressing

Prep Time: 15 minutes • Total Time: 35 minutes • **Makes 4 servings**

2 tablespoons extra-virgin olive oil, divided

1 small serrano chile pepper, seeded and diced (wear plastic gloves when handling)

1 small red onion, diced

1 can (14.5 ounces) pinto beans, rinsed and drained

4 organic corn tortillas

1 avocado, diced

½ small head cabbage, shredded

½ cup cilantro, chopped

Dressing

2 tablespoons freshly squeezed orange juice

3 tablespoons olive oil

1 clove garlic, minced

½ teaspoon ground coriander

¼ teaspoon ground cumin

1 teaspoon honey

⅛ teaspoon crushed red-pepper flakes

1. In a large skillet over medium heat, heat ½ tablespoon of the oil. Add the pepper and onion and cook for about 2 minutes. Add the beans and cook for 3 to 5 minutes, or until heated through. Remove the skillet from the heat and place the beans in a large bowl. Set aside.

2. Wipe the skillet clean and return it to medium heat. Add the remaining oil. Cook each tortilla for about 3 minutes per side, or until each side is slightly browned.

3. To the beans, add the avocado, cabbage, and cilantro. Gently stir to combine.

4. **TO MAKE THE DRESSING:** Combine the orange juice, oil, garlic, coriander, cumin, honey, and pepper flakes. Stir until well mixed. Drizzle over the beans.

5. Scoop one-quarter of the bean mixture onto each tortilla, fold up like a taco, and enjoy!

TIP: For added crunch, serve over a bed of salad greens instead of the tortilla.

Per serving: 366 calories, 24 g total fat, 4 g saturated fat, 34 g carbohydrates, 10 g dietary fiber, 7 g protein, 222 mg sodium

Grilled Fish Tacos with Slaw

Prep Time: 10 minutes + marinating time • Total Time: 25 minutes
• **Makes 4 servings**

Slaw

   6 cups finely sliced green and red cabbage
   1 cup chopped cilantro
   3 tablespoons freshly squeezed lime juice
   2 tablespoons olive oil
   1 tablespoon raw honey
   2 teaspoons ground cumin
   1½ teaspoons sea salt
   1½ teaspoons ground black pepper

Tacos

   1½ pounds firm white-fleshed fish fillets or steaks
       (Chilean sea bass, swordfish, or tilapia)
   ⅓ cup freshly squeezed lime juice
   8 organic corn tortillas (6" diameter)
   ½ cup salsa of choice
   1 avocado, sliced
   ½ cup whole milk plain yogurt (optional)

1. TO MAKE THE SLAW: In a large bowl, combine the cabbage and cilantro. In a small bowl, whisk together the lime juice, oil, honey, cumin, salt, and pepper. Pour over the cabbage slaw, toss, and chill.

2. TO MAKE THE TACOS: Rinse the fish, pat dry, and place in a large resealable plastic bag or glass dish. Pour the lime juice over the fish. Marinate in the refrigerator for at least 1 hour and up to 4 hours.

3. Coat a grill rack with cooking spray. Preheat the grill to medium-high. Drain the fish. Discard the marinade.

4. Grill the fish, turning once, for about 10 minutes, or until it flakes easily and is lightly browned on the outside. Transfer to a platter and let stand for 5 minutes. Cut into chunks.

5. Heat the tortillas on the grill for 10 to 15 seconds, turning once. Keep them soft; do not overcook.

6. Assemble each taco with fish, slaw, 1 tablespoon of the salsa, avocado slices, and 1 tablespoon of yogurt, if using.

Per serving: 473 calories, 18 g total fat, 4 g saturated fat, 42 g carbohydrates, 9 g dietary fiber, 38 g protein, 996 mg sodium

Seared Tuna
with Minted Quinoa Salad

Prep Time: 10 minutes • Total Time: 25 minutes • Makes 4 servings

- 1 cup quinoa, rinsed well and drained
- 2 cups water
- 1 teaspoon sea salt, divided
- 4 tuna steaks, about 6 ounces each
- 2 tablespoons coconut oil, melted, divided
- Peel of 1 lime
- 2 tablespoons lime juice
- 2 teaspoons chopped fresh cilantro
- ½ teaspoon coarsely ground black pepper
- 1 cucumber, cut in half, seeded, and diced
- ½ cup mint (about 1 handful), chopped
- 1 mango, diced (optional)
- 1 teaspoon honey

1. In a medium saucepan, combine the quinoa, water, and ½ teaspoon of the salt. Bring to a boil. Reduce the heat, cover, and simmer for 15 minutes. Remove from the heat and steam 5 minutes more, then remove the lid and fluff the quinoa with a fork.

2. While the quinoa cooks, rinse the tuna and pat dry with a paper towel. Rub with 1 tablespoon of the coconut oil and set aside.

3. In a small bowl, combine the lime peel, lime juice, cilantro, the remaining ½ teaspoon salt, and pepper.

4. In a medium bowl, combine the cucumber, mint, and mango, if using. Drizzle with the honey and stir. Add the cooked quinoa and gently stir to combine.

5. In a heavy-bottom or cast-iron skillet, heat the remaining 1 tablespoon coconut oil over medium-high heat. Place the oiled tuna in the skillet, being careful to avoid any splattering oil. Sear for 2 minutes, then carefully turn and sear for 2 minutes, or until the fish is just opaque (or to desired doneness). Serve the tuna on 4 plates and immediately pour the lime juice mixture over the tuna. Serve with the quinoa salad.

Per serving: 421 calories, 11 g total fat, 7 g saturated fat, 32 g carbohydrates, 5 g dietary fiber, 47 g protein, 466 mg sodium

Foil-Wrapped Fish with Olive Vegetable Medley

Prep Time: 15 minutes • Total Time: 30 minutes • Makes 4 servings

    4 fillets (1½ pounds) wild-caught fish (salmon, halibut, cod)
    ½ teaspoon sea salt
    ½ teaspoon ground black pepper
    3 tablespoons olive oil, divided
    1 lemon, cut into 4 slices
    2 cloves garlic, minced
    2 turnips, peeled and cut into ½" cubes
    2 heads broccoli, cut into small florets
    2 cups chopped kale
    2 carrots, cut into ½" pieces
    ¼ cup olive juice
  6–8 kalamata olives, pitted and sliced (optional)

1. Preheat the oven to 425°F.

2. Clean and pat the fish dry, removing any bones and skin, if needed. Sprinkle with the salt and pepper. Tear off 4 large pieces of foil and brush the centers of each piece with oil.

3. Place 1 piece of seasoned fish on each sheet of foil and top with a lemon slice. Drizzle 1 teaspoon of the oil over each fillet. Gather the foil up the sides of the fish and fold closed at the top to form a sealed packet. Set the packets on a baking sheet and bake for 12 minutes, or until the fish flakes easily.

4. Meanwhile, in a large skillet with a tight-fitting lid, heat the remaining oil over medium heat. Add the garlic and cook 1 minute. Add the turnips, broccoli, kale, carrots, olive juice, and olives (if using).

5. Cover the skillet and shake gently to ensure even cooking. Steam for 7 minutes, then taste for doneness and seasoning. Enjoy the vegetables with the fish.

Per serving: 510 calories, 24 g total fat, 4 g saturated fat, 32 g carbohydrates, 11 g dietary fiber, 48 g protein, 690 mg sodium

Roasted Shrimp and Broccoli with Couscous

Prep Time: 10 minutes • Total Time: 30 minutes • **Makes 4 servings**

- **1 pound broccoli crowns, cut into small florets**
- **¼ teaspoon red-pepper flakes**
- **¼ cup olive oil, divided**
- **¾ teaspoon sea salt, divided**
- **½ teaspoon ground black pepper, divided**
- **1 pound wild shrimp, peeled and deveined**
- **4 tablespoons lemon juice**
- **1 teaspoon lemon peel (optional)**
- **2 cups cooked couscous, warmed**

1. Preheat the oven to 425°F. Toss together the broccoli, pepper flakes, 2 tablespoons of the oil, and half of the salt and pepper.
2. In a separate bowl, toss together the shrimp, lemon juice, lemon peel (if using), and the remaining oil, salt, and pepper.
3. On a baking sheet, spread the broccoli and roast for 10 minutes. Add the shrimp (or place on a separate baking sheet, if needed) and roast for 10 minutes, or until the shrimp is opaque, turning once to ensure even cooking. Season the shrimp and broccoli with more lemon juice, if desired, and serve over the warm, cooked couscous.

Per serving: 314 calories, 16 g total fat, 2 g saturated fat, 26 g carbohydrates, 5 g dietary fiber, 20 g protein, 891 mg sodium

Tzatziki Chicken
with Greek Salad

Prep Time: 2 hours 30 minutes (includes marinating time) • Total Time: 3 hours
• Makes 5 servings

Tzatziki Chicken

- 1 cup whole milk plain yogurt (dairy-free option: 1 cup coconut milk)
- 4 cloves garlic, minced
- ½ teaspoon ground coriander
- 2 tablespoons lemon juice
- 2 teaspoons lemon peel
- ½ cup chopped mint
- ¼ teaspoon cracked black pepper
- 1 teaspoon sea salt
- 5 chicken breasts (6 ounces each, ¾" thick)

Greek Salad

- 2 cups cherry tomatoes, halved
- 1 English cucumber, diced
- 1 small yellow bell pepper, seeded and diced
- ½ red onion, diced
- ¼ cup kalamata olives, pitted and halved
- ¼ cup crumbled feta cheese
- ¼ cup chopped fresh Italian parsley
- 2 tablespoons olive oil
- 4 tablespoons lemon juice
- 1 teaspoon dried oregano
- ½ teaspoon Dijon mustard
- 1 clove garlic, minced
- ⅛ teaspoon sea salt
- ⅛ teaspoon ground black pepper

1. **TO MAKE THE CHICKEN:** Place the chicken in a glass baking dish. In a small bowl, mix the yogurt or coconut milk, garlic, coriander, lemon juice, lemon peel, mint, cracked pepper, and salt. Pour the marinade over the chicken and coat well. Marinate in the refrigerator for at least 2 hours or overnight.

2. Coat a grill rack or baking sheet with cooking spray. Preheat the grill to medium-high or the oven to 375°F. Grill the chicken for about 5 minutes per side, or bake the chicken for approximately 25 minutes, until a thermometer inserted in the thickest portion registers 170°F and the juices run clear.

3. **TO MAKE THE SALAD:** In a large bowl, toss the tomatoes, cucumber, bell pepper, onion, olives, cheese, and parsley. In a small bowl, whisk together the oil, lemon juice, oregano, mustard, garlic, salt, and black pepper. Pour the dressing over the salad mixture and stir to coat. Season with the salt and pepper as desired. Cover and refrigerate while preparing the chicken.

4. Serve each chicken breast with 1 cup of the Greek Salad.

TIP: This recipe is great as leftover for lunch the next day, as the flavors will meld overnight and only improve!

Per serving (1 chicken breast + 1 cup salad): 294 calories, 15 g total fat, 4 g saturated fat, 13 g carbohydrates, 3 g dietary fiber, 29 g protein, 698 mg sodium

Herbed Chicken and Barley with Dried Cherries and Pine Nuts

Prep Time: 4 hours (includes marinating time) • Total Time: 4 hours 15 minutes • **Makes 4 servings**

2 boneless, skinless chicken breasts

4 tablespoons + 2 teaspoons extra-virgin olive oil, divided

2 tablespoons fresh oregano or thyme

2 cloves garlic, minced

1 tablespoon Dijon mustard

3 tablespoons finely chopped shallots

2½ cups water, divided

⅓ cup Champagne or rice vinegar

½ teaspoon sea salt

¾ cup pearled barley

3 tablespoon freshly squeezed lemon juice

¼ teaspoon ground black pepper

½ cup dried cherries, chopped

½ cup toasted pine nuts, chopped

¼ cup fresh thyme

1. Place the chicken breasts in a resealable plastic bag or glass dish with 2 tablespoons of the oil and the oregano or thyme, garlic, and mustard. Marinate in the refrigerator for at least 4 hours.

2. Heat 2 teaspoons of the oil in a large saucepan over medium-high heat. Add the shallots and cook for 2 minutes, or until tender. Add 2 cups of the water and the vinegar and salt to the pan; bring to a boil. Add the barley. Reduce the heat, cover, and simmer for 40 minutes, or until the liquid is absorbed and the barley is tender. Remove the pan from the heat. Fluff the barley with a fork and set aside.

3. In a large bowl, whisk together the remaining 2 tablespoons oil with the lemon juice and pepper. Add the barley, cherries, pine nuts, and thyme and toss until coated with the dressing.

4. Coat a grill rack with cooking spray or oil. Preheat the grill to medium-high heat. Remove the chicken from the marinade. Discard the marinade. Grill the chicken for 4 minutes, turn, and cook for 4 minutes, or until a thermometer inserted in the thickest portion registers 165°F and the juices run clear. Remove the chicken and let stand for 5 minutes.

5. Slice the chicken. Place 1 cup cooked barley on each plate and top with chicken slices.

TIP: For extra greens, serve with a side salad.

Per serving: 554 calories, 31 g total fat, 4 g saturated fat, 47 g carbohydrates, 11 g dietary fiber, 25 g protein, 395 mg sodium

Lemon-Garlic Chicken and Polenta with Roasted Vegetables

Prep Time: 55 minutes (includes marinating time) • Total Time: 1 hour 35 minutes • **Makes 4 servings**

- 4 cloves garlic, minced
- 3 tablespoons lemon juice
- ⅓ cup olive oil, divided
- 4 boneless, skinless chicken breasts
- 1 small eggplant, peeled and cut into ¼" slices
- 1 small zucchini, cut into ¼" slices
- 1 small yellow squash, cut into ¼" slices
- 6 mushrooms, sliced
- 1 red bell pepper, seeded and cut into strips
- 4 cups low-sodium organic vegetable broth
- 2 cups water
- ¼ teaspoon sea salt, divided
- 1½ cups coarse polenta (corn grits)
- 2 tablespoons butter
- ½ teaspoon cracked black pepper, divided
- 6 dry-packed sun-dried tomatoes
- 10 ounces frozen spinach, thawed and squeezed dry
- 2 plum tomatoes, sliced
- 8 olives, pitted and chopped
- 2 teaspoons fresh oregano, chopped

1. In a small bowl, whisk together the garlic, lemon juice, and 3 tablespoons of the oil. Place the chicken in a resealable plastic bag or glass dish and pour in the garlic marinade. Marinate in the refrigerator for 30 minutes to 1 hour.

2. Coat a broiler-pan rack or grill rack with cooking spray. Preheat the broiler or grill. Position the rack 4" from the heat source.

3. On the prepared rack, arrange the eggplant, zucchini, squash, mushrooms, and bell pepper in a single layer and brush with 2 tablespoons of the oil. Cook until soft, turning as needed, about 4 minutes. Remove the vegetables from the heat, cool, and chop into chunks.

4. Preheat the oven to 350°F. Coat a casserole or baking dish with olive oil cooking spray.

5. In a large saucepan, bring the broth, water, and $\frac{1}{8}$ teaspoon of the salt to a boil. Reduce the heat and slowly whisk in the polenta. Cover and cook for about 15 minutes, stirring occasionally. When the polenta comes away from the side of the pan, stir in the butter and season with $\frac{1}{4}$ teaspoon of the black pepper. Remove from the heat.

6. Spread the polenta into the prepared casserole or baking dish and brush with the remaining 1 teaspoon oil. Bake for 10 to 15 minutes. Remove and keep warm.

7. Meanwhile, place the sun-dried tomatoes in a small bowl and cover with hot water. Set aside to rehydrate, about 10 minutes. Drain, then chop.

8. Spread the drained spinach over the polenta. Layer on the plum tomatoes, sun-dried tomatoes, and olives. Top with the roasted vegetables. Sprinkle with the oregano and the remaining salt and pepper. Return to the oven for 10 minutes.

9. Coat another broiler-pan or grill rack with cooking spray. Preheat the broiler or the grill to medium-high heat. Remove the chicken from the marinade. Discard the marinade. Place the chicken on the rack and cook for 4 to 5 minutes on each side, or until a thermometer inserted in the thickest portion registers 165°F and the juices run clear. Remove from the heat and set aside.

10. When the polenta is warmed through, remove from the oven, cut into wedges, and serve with the chicken.

Per serving: 691 calories, 28 g total fat, 7 g saturated fat, 64 g carbohydrates, 12 g dietary fiber, 48 g protein, 689 mg sodium

Brined Chicken Breast with Roasted Broccoli

Prep Time: 1 hour 5 minutes (includes brining time) • Total Time: 1 hour 25 minutes
• **Makes 4 servings**

> 3 **cups water**
> 2 **tablespoons + ½ teaspoon sea salt**
> 1 **pound boneless, skinless chicken breasts (about 2 large)**
> 2 **tablespoons olive oil, divided**
> 1 **head broccoli, stalk chopped into 2" pieces, leaving florets whole**
> 1 **tablespoon balsamic vinegar**

1. Pour the water and 2 tablespoons of the salt into a medium-size bowl and add the chicken. Let the chicken brine for 1 hour, then remove the breasts, rinse, and pat dry with paper towels.
2. Place each chicken breast on a piece of plastic wrap and fold the plastic over it. Using a rolling pin, lightly pound the thickest portion of chicken until the entire breast is nearly the same thickness, about ½" to ¾" thick.
3. Heat ½ tablespoon of the oil in a skillet on medium heat. Place the chicken in the skillet and cook for about 5 minutes per side, flipping halfway through, until each side is nicely browned, or until a thermometer inserted in the center registers 165°F and the chicken is no longer pink. Place the chicken on a cutting board and slice into strips.
4. Meanwhile, roast the broccoli. Preheat the oven to 400°F. In a medium-size bowl, toss the chopped broccoli in the remaining oil and the vinegar.
5. On a baking sheet, spread the broccoli evenly and sprinkle with the remaining ½ teaspoon salt. Place the sheet in the oven on the middle rack. Cook for 12 minutes, or until the broccoli is golden and tender. Remove from the oven and serve with the chicken strips.

Per serving: 212 calories, 10 g total fat, 2 g saturated fat, 11 g carbohydrates, 4 g dietary fiber, 22 g protein, 514 mg sodium

Thai Green Curry Beef with Basmati Rice

Prep Time: 10 minutes • Total Time: 1 hour 10 minutes • Makes 4 servings

- 1 cup brown basmati rice
- 2¼ cups water
- ½ teaspoon sea salt
- 1 tablespoon canola oil
- 1 pound beef sirloin, cut into 1" cubes
- 3 tablespoons green curry paste
- 2 cans (14 ounces each) coconut milk (fat skimmed from top of each can)
- 1 tablespoon minced garlic
- 2 tablespoons minced fresh ginger
- 2 cups Napa cabbage or bok choy (½ small head), thinly sliced
- 1 red bell pepper, seeded and cut into thin strips
- 1 carrot, cut into thin 2" sticks
- 1 cup mushrooms, sliced
- Juice of 1 lime (optional)

1. In a large saucepan, bring the rice, water, and salt to a boil. Reduce the heat, cover, and simmer for 35 minutes, or until the rice is tender and the water has evaporated.

2. Heat the oil in a wide pot or wok on medium-high heat. Add the beef cubes and cook for 5 minutes, stirring often, until browned on all sides. Transfer to a plate. To the pot or wok, add the curry and the thick coconut milk (from the top parts of the cans) and bring to a boil, stirring until dissolved. Reduce the heat and simmer for 3 minutes.

3. Add the garlic, ginger, cabbage, bell pepper, carrot, and mushrooms and boil gently for 5 minutes, or until the vegetables are cooked but not mushy. Turn off the heat and add the lime juice, if using, and salt to taste. Serve with the rice.

TIP: Use just 2 tablespoons of the green curry paste for a milder dish.

Per serving: 562 calories, 27 g total fat, 18 g saturated fat, 47 g carbohydrates, 4 g dietary fiber, 31 g protein, 518 mg sodium

Red, White, and Blue Burgers with Creamy Coleslaw

Prep Time: 15 minutes • **Total Time: 30 minutes** • **Makes 4 servings**

Coleslaw

- ½ head green cabbage, thinly sliced
- ½ head red cabbage, thinly sliced
- 2 carrots, grated
- 1 beet, grated
- 3 scallions, thinly sliced
- 2 tablespoons apple cider vinegar
- 2 tablespoons olive oil
- ⅓ cup whole milk plain yogurt
- 2 teaspoons mustard seeds
- ½ teaspoon sea salt
- ½ teaspoon ground black pepper

Burgers

- 1 pound 90% lean grass-fed ground beef
- 3 cloves garlic, minced
- ½ onion, finely chopped
- ½ red bell pepper, seeded and finely chopped
- 2 tablespoons fresh thyme or 2 teaspoons dried
- 1 egg
- ¼ cup ground flaxseed (flaxseed meal)
- ⅓ cup crumbled blue cheese (optional)
- Ketchup, sweetened with agave or maple syrup, such as Organic Ville Ketchup (optional)
- 1 tomato, sliced
- 1 avocado, sliced
- ¼ teaspoon sea salt (sprinkle on top)
- ½ teaspoon ground black pepper (sprinkle on top)
- Large leaf salad greens (romaine, red or green leaf lettuce, or kale), washed
- 4 whole grain hamburger buns (optional)

1. **TO MAKE THE COLESLAW:** In a large salad bowl, toss together the cabbage, carrots, beet, and scallions. Set aside.

2. In a small bowl, whisk together the vinegar, oil, yogurt, mustard seeds, salt, and pepper. Pour the dressing over the coleslaw and toss. Refrigerate until serving. (This salad may be made a day in advance and stored in the refrigerator.)

3. **TO MAKE THE BURGERS:** Coat a grill rack with cooking spray. Preheat the grill to medium-high heat.

4. In a large bowl, combine the ground beef, garlic, onion, bell pepper, thyme, egg, flaxseed, and blue cheese (if using), massaging the ingredients together with your hands. Shape into 4 patties $\frac{1}{2}$" thick.

5. Place the patties on the prepared rack. Grill for 4 to 5 minutes on each side, or until a thermometer inserted in the center registers 160°F and the meat is no longer pink.

6. Top the burgers with ketchup (if using), a tomato slice, and avocado slices and sprinkle with the salt and pepper. Place each burger stack in the center of a large piece of lettuce or kale, leaving excess lettuce on 3 sides of the burger. Fold the bottom side of the lettuce up, then wrap the right and left sides over. Secure with a toothpick. Alternatively, place each burger with toppings in a hamburger bun. Serve with the coleslaw.

TIP: To save time, slice the coleslaw ingredients in a food processor.

Per serving (1¼-pound burger): 513 calories, 29 g total fat, 8 g saturated fat, 33 g carbohydrates, 13 g dietary fiber, 32 g protein, 504 mg sodium

Tzatziki Lamb Wraps

Prep Time: 10 minutes • Total Time: 25 minutes • **Makes 4 servings**

    1 cup water
    ½ cup quinoa, rinsed well and drained
    1¼ teaspoons sea salt, divided
    ½ cup brown rice flour
    1 tablespoon ground cumin
    1 teaspoon cinnamon
    ½ teaspoon allspice
    ½ teaspoon ground black pepper
    1 egg
    1 pound ground lamb
    7 scallions, thinly sliced, white and green parts divided
    2 tablespoon extra-virgin olive oil, divided
    1 cup whole milk plain yogurt (dairy-free option: 1 cup coconut milk)
    ¼ teaspoon red wine vinegar
    1 clove garlic, minced
    ½ cucumber, peeled, seeded, and diced
    1 tablespoon mint, chopped
    8 large butter lettuce leaves, rinsed and patted dry

1. In a saucepan, bring the water, quinoa, and ⅛ teaspoon of the salt to a boil. Reduce the heat and cook, covered, for 15 minutes. Remove the saucepan from the heat, fluff the quinoa with a fork, and set aside.

2. In a medium bowl, whisk together the flour, cumin, cinnamon, allspice, 1 teaspoon of the salt, and the pepper. Add the egg and mix until combined. Add the lamb and the white parts of the scallions. Using your hands, combine the ingredients. Add more flour, if needed, to hold the mixture together. Form into 1½" balls, pressing to flatten slightly before cooking.

3. In a cast-iron skillet over medium heat, heat 1 tablespoon of the oil. Add the lamb balls and brown for about 5 minutes on each side. Cover the skillet, reduce the heat to medium-low, and cook for 5 more minutes, or until the balls are no longer pink in the center.

4. In a medium-size bowl, combine the green parts of the scallions with the yogurt or coconut milk, vinegar, garlic, cucumber, and mint.

5. To serve, fill each lettuce leaf with 1 lamb ball and equal portions of quinoa and tzatziki (yogurt dressing). Fold each leaf to form either a wrap or lettuce cup.

Per serving: 613 calories, 39 g total fat, 15 g saturated fat, 37 g carbohydrates, 5 g dietary fiber, 28 g protein, 619 mg sodium

Pork Lettuce Cups

Prep Time: 1 hour (includes marinating time) • Total Time: 1 hour 15 minutes
• **Makes 4 servings**

  2 tablespoons tamari
  2 tablespoons balsamic vinegar
  4 cloves garlic, crushed
  2 tablespoons chopped fresh ginger
  2 tablespoons sweet chili sauce
  1 pound pork tenderloin, trimmed and cut into ½" pieces
3–4 tablespoons dark sesame oil
  ½ head bok choy, thinly shredded
  2 carrots, grated
  ¼ teaspoon sea salt
  ¼ teaspoon ground black pepper
  8 large butter lettuce leaves, rinsed and patted dry
  4 scallions, sliced into thin 2" strips
  1 cucumber, peeled and cut into thin 2" strips
  2 cups cooked short-grain brown rice, warmed

1. In a small bowl, whisk together the tamari, vinegar, garlic, ginger, and chili sauce. Pour into a large resealable plastic bag or glass dish and add the cut pork. Marinate in the refrigerator for 30 minutes to 4 hours.

2. Heat 3 tablespoons of the oil in a wok or skillet over high heat. Add the pork, marinade, bok choy, and carrots. Separate any pieces that might stick together. Cook without stirring for 1 minute. Turn and stir-fry for 2 minutes on the other side, until the pork is cooked through. (Add the remaining 1 tablespoon oil, if necessary.) Season with the salt and pepper. Spoon into a bowl.

3. To serve, fill 1 lettuce leaf at a time with 1 heaping tablespoon of the pork mixture, scallions, and cucumbers. To eat, pull all sides of the lettuce leaf together to form a pouch or bowl. Serve with the warm rice.

Per serving: 392 calories, 14 g total fat, 3 g saturated fat, 37 g carbohydrates, 5 g dietary fiber, 29 g protein, 783 mg sodium

Pan-Roasted Edamame

Prep Time: 10 minutes • Total Time: 20 minutes • **Makes 4 servings**

> 4 cups fresh or frozen edamame
> 1 tablespoon olive oil
> ½ teaspoon onion powder
> ½ teaspoon ground cumin
> ⅛ teaspoon cracked black pepper
> ½ teaspoon sea salt

1. Bring a large pot of water to a boil over high heat. Add the edamame and cook for about 5 minutes, or until bright green. Drain.

2. Heat the oil in a large nonstick skillet over medium-high heat. Add the onion powder and cumin and cook for 30 seconds, or until fragrant. Add the edamame and cook, tossing, for about 1 minute, or until hot and well coated. Add the pepper and salt and remove from the heat. Transfer to a bowl and serve warm or at room temperature.

Per serving: 162 calories, 9 g total fat, 0.5 g saturated fat, 11 g carbohydrates, 6 g dietary fiber, 12 g protein, 204 mg sodium

SNACKS

Spicy Chickpeas

Prep Time: 15 minutes • Total Time: 50 minutes • **Makes 8 servings**

> 2 cans (15 ounces each) chickpeas, rinsed, drained, and patted dry
>
> ¼ cup olive oil
>
> ½ teaspoon sea salt
>
> 1 teaspoon ground cumin
>
> ½ teaspoon smoked paprika
>
> ⅛ teaspoon ground red pepper

1. Preheat oven to 400°F.
2. In a bowl, thoroughly combine the chickpeas, oil, salt, cumin, paprika, and red pepper.
3. Spread the chickpeas in a single layer on a baking sheet and bake for 30 to 45 minutes, or until crunchy. Be careful not to burn.

TIP: Make these ahead of time and store in a sealed container in the refrigerator.

Per serving (about ⅓ cup): 123 calories, 8 g total fat, 1 g saturated fat, 9 g carbohydrates, 3 g dietary fiber, 3 g protein, 291 mg sodium

Crunchy Kale Chips

Prep Time: 5 minutes • Total Time: 10 minutes • **Makes 4 servings**

> 1 bunch lacinato or red Russian kale, rinsed and dried
>
> 1 tablespoon olive oil
>
> ½ teaspoon sea salt

1. Preheat the oven from 350°F to 375°F, depending on your oven. The kale chips burn quickly, so keep the temperature on the lower end if your oven runs high or has hot spots.

2. Remove the thick stem of the kale by folding each leaf in half lengthwise and cutting the center rib away. Make sure the kale is quite dry.

3. Pour the oil into a small bowl. Dip your fingers in the oil and rub some over each kale leaf, front and back.

4. Arrange the kale on several baking sheets, making sure not to crowd the leaves. Sprinkle the salt over the top. Bake for 5 to 7 minutes, keeping an eye on the chips to make sure they don't burn. Turn the chips over and bake for another 2 to 3 minutes. You may need more or less time, depending on your oven. The chips are ready when they are bright green; discard any brown ones, as they are burnt and will taste bitter.

Per serving: 86 calories, 5 g total fat, 0.5 g saturated fat, 10 g carbohydrates, 2 g dietary fiber, 5 g protein, 338 mg sodium

Toasted Walnut "Pâté"

Prep Time: 10 minutes • Total Time: 25 minutes • **Makes 8 servings**

- 1 tablespoon olive oil
- 1 cup walnuts
- 1 small onion, chopped
- 4 ounces mushrooms, sliced
- ½ teaspoon dried thyme
- 2 cloves garlic, minced
- 2 tablespoons freshly squeezed lemon juice
- 2 tablespoons chopped fresh parsley
- 1 teaspoon tamari
-    Ground black pepper

1. Heat the oil in a skillet over medium heat until it sizzles. Add the walnuts. Cook for 3 minutes, stirring occasionally, or until the nuts are toasted. Add the onion, mushrooms, and thyme. Cook, stirring, for 8 minutes, or until the onion is softened. Add the garlic. Stir just until the garlic is incorporated. Remove the skillet from the heat. Cool to room temperature.
2. Transfer the mixture to the bowl of a blender or a food processor fitted with a metal blade. Process, scraping the bowl as needed, for about 3 minutes, or until a coarse paste forms. Add the lemon juice, parsley, tamari, and pepper to taste. Pulse until just combined. Serve immediately or refrigerate for up to 1 week.

TIP: Serve with carrots, apple slices, whole grain crackers, or rice cakes for a protein-packed snack.

Per serving: 106 calories, 10 g total fat, 1 g saturated fat, 4 g carbohydrates, 1 g dietary fiber, 3 g protein, 41 mg sodium

Danish Cheese Pie

Prep Time: 35 minutes • **Total Time:** 1 hour 40 minutes • **Makes 8 servings**

Piecrust

- 1 cup ground raw almonds (almond flour can be used for up to ½ cup of this)
- ½ cup almond flour
- Pinch of sea salt
- Pinch of cinnamon
- 1 tablespoon coconut oil, melted to a liquid
- 1 egg, beaten

Pie Filling

- 1 cup chopped dates
- 2 tablespoons orange juice
- 1 teaspoon grated orange peel
- 1 container (15 ounces) whole ricotta cheese
- 1 tablespoon honey
- 2 eggs, well beaten
- ¼ cup full-fat canned coconut milk
- 2 tablespoons almond flour
- 1 teaspoon almond extract
- Dash of nutmeg
- Dash of cinnamon

1. **TO MAKE THE CRUST:** Preheat the oven to 350°F.
2. In a large bowl, mix together the ground almonds, almond flour, salt, and cinnamon. In a small bowl, mix together the melted oil and beaten egg. Add the wet ingredients to the dry and stir the dough with a rubber spatula until thoroughly combined.
3. Turn the dough into a 9" pie plate or tart pan. Flatten and press the dough evenly, so that you have a uniform thickness across the bottom and edges of the pan. Bake for 5 to 7 minutes on the middle rack of the oven. Remove the crust from the oven and let cool before filling.

4. **TO MAKE THE FILLING:** Preheat the oven to 400°F.

5. In a shallow dish, soak the dates in just enough boiling water to cover for 10 minutes. Add the dates and the soaking water to a food processor and puree until a paste forms. Add the orange juice and orange peel and process. Add the ricotta cheese and puree until smooth. Add the honey, eggs, coconut milk, almond flour, and almond extract. Pulse to combine.

6. Pour into the baked and cooled crust. Lightly sprinkle with the nutmeg and cinnamon.

7. Bake for 10 minutes, reduce the heat to 350°F, and bake for 30 minutes until firm. Cool and serve. This is great served with a sweet fresh fruit like peaches or berries.

Variations:

The filling can be baked in little single-serving ramekins as a custard, without crust.

This crust is also excellent filled with coconut ice cream and fresh fruit.

TIP: Use a crust shield during baking to prevent burnt edges. If you don't have a shield, foil works well: Cut a circle the size of the filling out of a piece of foil. Lay the sheet of foil (with the circle removed) over the crust edges so the filling is uncovered but the crust is protected from direct oven heat.

Per serving: 382 calories, 25 g total fat, 9 g saturated fat, 26 g carbohydrates, 4 g dietary fiber, 15 g protein, 76 mg sodium

Protein Power "Barre"

Prep Time: 15 minutes • Total Time: 1 hour 15 minutes • **Makes 10 servings**

6 dried figs

2 tablespoons coconut oil

¼ cup sunflower butter or almond butter

¼ cup dried cranberries

¼ cup coconut flakes

¼ cup almond meal

Pinch of ground cinnamon

⅛ teaspoon sea salt (omit if the sunflower or almond butter is salted)

1 cup pecans

¼ cup dark chocolate chips

1. In a food processor, combine the figs, coconut oil and sunflower or almond butter. Process until blended. Add the cranberries, coconut, almond meal, cinnamon, and salt (if using), and process until the mixture is well incorporated. It's okay if it's a bit chunky at this point. Add the pecans and chocolate chips and pulse until the mixture looks like cookie dough.

2. Transfer the "dough" into an 8" × 8" baking dish and press the mixture down flat with the back of a spoon.

3. Store in the fridge for at least 1 hour to harden. Cut into bars for grab-and-go snacking. Store extras in the refrigerator for up to 1 week.

Per serving: 228 calories, 18 g total fat, 6 g saturated fat, 16 g carbohydrates, 4 g dietary fiber, 4 g protein, 16 mg sodium

Chocolate-Hazelnut Bites

Prep Time: 25 minutes • Total Time: 55 minutes • **Makes 12 servings**

> 1 cup pitted Medjool dates
> 1½ cups roasted hazelnuts
> ¼ cup unsweetened cocoa powder
> 2 tablespoons almond butter
> 1 tablespoon coconut butter
> ½ teaspoon orange extract
> ½ teaspoon almond extract
> ¼ teaspoon sea salt
> 2 tablespoons finely shredded unsweetened coconut

1. Soak the dates in a bowl of hot water until soft, about 20 minutes. Drain.
2. In a food processor, combine the drained dates, hazelnuts, cocoa powder, almond butter, coconut butter, extracts, and salt. Process for 2 minutes, or until the mixture is finely ground and holds together when pressed. You may need to add a little water.
3. Scoop out rounded spoonfuls of dough with a mini-ice-cream scoop (2 tablespoons). Press the dough in your palms to make a ball. Roll that ball in the shredded coconut.
4. Place the finished balls on a plate or baking sheet or in a glass storage container. Refrigerate for an hour or so before eating. Store in the freezer or fridge.

Per serving (2 pieces): 170 calories, 13 g total fat, 2 g saturated fat, 14 g carbohydrates, 4 g dietary fiber, 4 g protein, 39 mg sodium

Avocado-Coconut Ice Cream

Prep Time: 10 minutes • Total Time: 1 hour 25 minutes (plus additional freezing time) • **Makes 4 servings**

3 Hass avocados, flesh scooped out

1 can (13.5 ounces) coconut milk

1 cup whole milk plain Greek yogurt

⅓ cup maple syrup

1 tablespoon vanilla extract

⅓ cup cacao nibs

⅓ cup shredded unsweetened coconut

1. In a food processor, puree the avocados until smooth.

2. Add the coconut milk, yogurt, syrup, and vanilla. Process for 2 to 3 minutes, or until completely smooth.

3. Transfer the mixture to a bowl, cover, and refrigerate for 1 to 2 hours, or until thoroughly chilled.

4. Process the mixture in an ice-cream maker according to the manufacturer's instructions. A couple of minutes before the mixture has finished churning, add the cacao nibs and coconut. For soft-serve ice cream, serve at once. If a firmer texture is desired, freeze overnight. Let stand at room temperature for about 15 minutes before serving.

Per serving: 650 calories, 54 g total fat, 33 g saturated fat, 37 g carbohydrates, 12 g dietary fiber, 9 g protein, 43 mg sodium

Sadie's Strawberry Shake

Prep Time: 5 minutes • Total Time: 10 minutes • **Makes 2 servings**

2 cups whole milk Greek yogurt

10 pitted dates (no more than 3 ounces)

1 cup strawberries (fresh are best, but frozen work)

1 teaspoon vanilla extract

2 cups ice

In a blender or food processor, combine the yogurt, dates, strawberries, vanilla, and ice. Enjoy.

Per serving: 349 calories, 11 g total fat, 8 g saturated fat, 41 g carbohydrates, 4 g dietary fiber, 21 g protein, 73 mg sodium

Chapter 8

The 7-DAY BODY BONUS

I DESIGNED THIS SPECIAL 7-DAY BONUS PLAN FOR TIMES WHEN YOU want to jump-start your energy and weight-loss goals and feel good fast. I do this program before important events when I need to be on my A game, like weddings, reunions, or anything that involves a bathing suit! This program is the perfect way to bounce back after vacations or holidays, when you may have fallen off the wagon and need a boost back to your healthy lifestyle. You can do this program during or after the basic Love Your Lower Body plan or on its own to turbocharge your weight loss.

You will follow an exercise plan that is based on the Love Your Lower Body workouts. It is designed to keep you moving all day long—because when you move more, you burn more calories and sustain your energy levels.

Each day, you will have one of my favorite smoothies for breakfast, a salad or leftovers for lunch, and a balanced dinner. The goal is to keep your meal plan clean and simple. There is no gluten, dairy, sugar, alcohol, or grains in your diet this week. Yes, you'll need to part with your nightly glass of wine. And yes, you'll need to forgo your morning coffee with hazelnut creamer. But, trust me, you won't need them. You can do this!

All of your meals emphasize foods that are designed to cleanse your body, fueling weight loss and restoring energy. You will notice that many of the recipes are vegan, but you are welcome to add lean animal protein such as eggs, grilled chicken, or fish to each meal for extra protein if you need to go beyond plant-based protein sources.

On the following pages, you will find the 7-Day Body Bonus Workout Challenge and Diet Challenge instructions, including a fun new move and six refreshing and fueling smoothie recipes. Ready? Let's get started!

7-Day Body Bonus Workout Challenge

On Days 1 through 5, you will exercise for a total of 60 minutes.

Morning Wake-Up

- 10 Transformative Minutes (page 98)
- Standing Stretch (page 99)
- Mat Workout (page 160)
- Mat Stretch (page 161)

Total: 30 minutes

Power Lunch

- Full-Body Blast (page 131)
- Standing Stretch (page 99)

Total: 15 minutes

Evening Express

- Full-Body Blast (page 131)
- Mat Stretch (page 161)

Total: 15 minutes

DAILY TOTAL: 60 MINUTES

Additionally, every day you'll choose one or two of these moves to use as barre3 Boosts. Do them for a minute each.

- Horse Pose Pliés (page 100)
- Push-Pulls (page 190)
- Sumo Squats (page 112)
- Starfish: 1 minute per side (page 104)
- Plank Jacks (see facing page)

To see a sample schedule, turn to page 292.

NEW! Plank Jacks

SETUP: Start in a Plank position at the barre. Your body is in line from your heels to your head with your core drawing in and your spine in neutral. Your hands are a bit wider than your shoulders. Hold for 1 minute.

MOVEMENT 1: Gently jump your feet out wider than your hips, landing with softly bent knees.

MOVEMENT 2: Gently jump your feet into your Plank position.

MODIFICATION: To increase the challenge, do Plank on the floor.

Plank Jacks are an efficient way to elevate the heart rate, burn calories, and get all the core benefits of Plank in one exercise.

Do these on a sturdy surface like a wall-mounted counter or kitchen island.

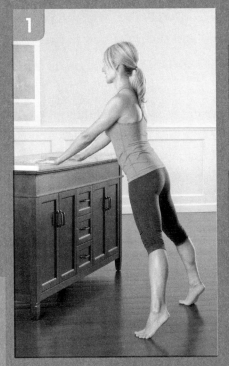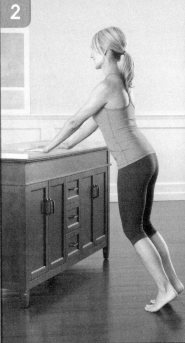

RANGE: Large
REPS: 30
TIME: 1 minute

Body Bonus Diet Challenge

This 7-day meal plan will help you slim down fast. The plan shows plenty of variety, but feel free to repeat meals. For example, on busy days, I will have a smoothie for breakfast, lunch, and snack! If you make a big batch of soup, you can have it for multiple meals as well.

In place of grains, add even more dark green leafy vegetables into your meals. Remember to always include in each meal and snack a protein (like nuts and legumes), healthy fats (like avocado, olive oil, and seeds), and fiber (this week, focus on veggies and especially leafy greens).

Body Bonus Tips

- Refer to the Portion Prescription on page 46 to ensure your meals are balanced and the right size to fuel your success.

- When hunger strikes between meals, it might actually mean you need more water. Keep refilling your water bottle all day long.

- Power your success with social media. Some of my clients with the best weight-loss results use Facebook, Twitter, and other social media sites to share their progress daily and get positive feedback from their online community.

Your Eats for the Week

You'll enjoy a smoothie for breakfast each day.

For lunch and dinner, choose grainless options from the recipes in Chapter 7 and be sure to include plenty of lean protein.

Select one or two snacks per day from this list.

- Leftover smoothie (my favorite snack—it is so easy to save some to sip on later in the day)

- Handful of nuts

- 2 tablespoons nut butter with ½ sliced apple

- 2 tablespoons hummus with ½ cup veggies

See page 292 for a sample menu.

Sadie's Favorite "Sneaky Greens" Smoothies

For breakfast, choose from one of my favorite "sneaky greens" smoothies below or prepare your own smoothie using my DIY Smoothie guide on page 226. Just combine your chosen ingredients in a high-speed blender for 1 to 2 minutes, or until well blended, and enjoy!

Citrus Avocado Smoothie

- 1 whole grapefruit, peeled
- 1 cup spinach
- ½ avocado
- 1 tablespoon maple syrup
- 2 tablespoons fresh mint
- 1 cup almond milk
- 2 tablespoons ground flaxseed
- 2 tablespoons hemp seeds
- 1 cup ice

Hemp Berry Smoothie

- 1 cup water
- 1 cup hemp milk
- 1 cup kale
- ½ cup blueberries
- ½ cup strawberries
- 2 tablespoons hemp seeds
- 2 tablespoons chia seeds
- 5 pitted dates
- 1 cup ice

Berry Green Smoothie

- 1 cup water
- 1 cup almond milk
- 2 cups spinach
- 2 tablespoons ground flaxseed
- 2 tablespoons hemp seeds
- ½ frozen banana
- 1 cup frozen boysenberries
- ½ teaspoon cinnamon
- ½ teaspoon vanilla
- 1 cup ice

PB & Banana Smoothie

- 1 cup water
- 1 cup almond milk
- 1 cup spinach
- ¼ cup peanut butter
- 1 banana
- 2 tablespoons ground flaxseed
- 1 teaspoon vanilla
- ½ teaspoon cinnamon
- 4 pitted dates
- 1 cup ice

Pineapple Paradise Smoothie

- 1 cup water
- 1 cup coconut water
- 1 cup pineapple chunks
- 1 cup spinach
- ¼ cup Brazil nuts
- 2 tablespoons ground flaxseed
- 2 tablespoons chia seeds
- 1 cup ice

Chocolate Cherry Smoothie

- 1 cup water
- 1 cup almond milk
- 1 cup pitted cherries (frozen work great)
- ¼ cup almond butter
- 1 tablespoon raw cacao powder
- 1 cup spinach
- 5 pitted dates
- 1 cup ice

YOUR 7-DAY BODY

WORKOUT	DAY 1	DAY 2	DAY 3
This is a week to push your limits, but remember to listen to your body, too, taking breaks and modifying as needed.	10 Transformative Minutes, Standing Stretch, Mat Workout, and Mat Stretch (30 min) + Full-Body Blast and Standing Stretch (15 min) + Full-Body Blast and Mat Stretch (15 min) + 1–2 barre3 Boosts (1–2 min)	10 Transformative Minutes, Standing Stretch, Mat Workout, and Mat Stretch (30 min) + Full-Body Blast and Standing Stretch (15 min) + Full-Body Blast and Mat Stretch (15 min) + 1–2 barre3 Boosts (1–2 min)	1–2 barre3 Boosts (1–2 min)

MENU	DAY 1	DAY 2	DAY 3
BREAKFAST	Citrus Avocado Smoothie (page 291)	Berry Green Smoothie (page 291)	Pineapple Paradise Smoothie (page 291)
SNACK(S)	Handful of almonds	1 Tbsp peanut butter with ½ sliced apple	2 Tbsp hummus with ½ cup cauliflower
LUNCH	DIY Salad and Dressing (page 240)	Spicy Harvest Soup leftovers from last night's dinner	Black Bean Bowls with Cumin-Lime Dressing leftovers from last night's dinner *Serve over greens.*
DINNER	Spicy Harvest Soup (page 238) *Use avocado in place of the sour cream garnish.*	Black Bean Bowls with Cumin-Lime Dressing (page 244) *Replace the quinoa with mixed greens and serve as a salad.*	Rough-Chopped Salad with Chicken and Pistachio-Herb Vinaigrette (page 248) *To make vegan, omit the chicken and add your favorite plant-based protein, such as nuts or legumes.*

Chart your progress. Place a checkmark for each day you stay on plan!

I ATE ON PLAN			
I EXERCISED ON PLAN			

BONUS PLAN

DAY 4	DAY 5	DAY 6	DAY 7
10 Transformative Minutes, Standing Stretch, Mat Workout, and Mat Stretch (30 min)	10 Transformative Minutes, Standing Stretch, Mat Workout, and Mat Stretch (30 min)	10 Transformative Minutes, Standing Stretch, Mat Workout, and Mat Stretch (30 min)	1–2 barre3 Boosts (1–2 min)
+	+	+	
Full-Body Blast and Standing Stretch (15 min)	Full-Body Blast and Standing Stretch (15 min)	Full-Body Blast and Standing Stretch (15 min)	
+	+	+	
Full-Body Blast and Mat Stretch (15 min)	Full-Body Blast and Mat Stretch (15 min)	Full-Body Blast and Mat Stretch (15 min)	
+	+	+	
1–2 barre3 Boosts (1–2 min)	1–2 barre3 Boosts (1–2 min)	1–2 barre3 Boosts (1–2 min)	

DAY 4	DAY 5	DAY 6	DAY 7
PB & Banana Smoothie (page 291)	Hemp Berry Smoothie (page 291)	Chocolate Cherry Smoothie (page 291)	DIY Smoothie (page 291)
Leftover smoothie Handful of pistachios	1 Tbsp almond butter with ½ sliced apple	Leftover smoothie Handful of walnuts	2 Tbsp hummus with ½ cup baby carrots
DIY Salad and Dressing	Black Bean Chili leftovers from last night's dinner	DIY Salad and Dressing	Mediterranean Quinoa Salad with Carrot Fries leftovers from last night's dinner
Black Bean Chili (page 257)	DIY Salad and Dressing	Mediterranean Quinoa Salad with Carrot Fries (page 243) *Omit the quinoa and serve with as much spinach as you like.*	Foil-Wrapped Fish with Olive Vegetable Medley (page 262) *To make vegan, replace the fish with tofu.*

Raising the Barre

JENNIFER DASHNEY-LONGBINE

AGE: 34   POUNDS LOST: 13.6   INCHES LOST: 9½ *including 5½ from her waist*

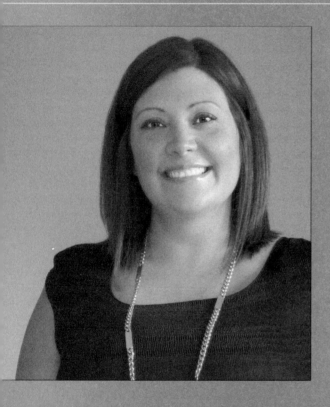

I was thin most of my life. In fact, in my late teens I even modeled for a while. But at age 22, I faced cervical cancer, followed by ongoing health issues ranging from kidney complications to an irregular heartbeat. By age 30, I had gone from a super-thin 120 pounds to more than 250. I was also diagnosed with polycystic ovarian syndrome, which helped explain in part why I struggled to lose weight. I felt like my health was out of control. Then, at my heaviest, against all odds I became pregnant with twins. They came early—at 33.5 weeks. As they fought for survival in the NICU, I couldn't help but think that my poor health had affected theirs.

I had a lot of time to think during the next couple of months as I recovered from my C-section and breastfed the boys. I thought about what kind of mother, wife, and woman I wanted to be. I decided that it was time to make some long-overdue changes. I did a detox with the support of my naturopath to lose the first 40 pounds. Over the next 2 years, I slowly kept losing, learning about my gluten intolerance and being mindful of my diet. By January 2013, I was ready to focus on fitness. At that point, I had about 50 pounds left to lose to get to the goal weight my doctor had set for me.

I tried barre3 for a little while last year and although I fell off the wagon, I saw some light at the end of the tunnel. When I got into the test panel, I was excited. In just 8 weeks, I've experienced a complete shift in preferences. I now genuinely prefer whole foods. I look forward to my workouts. I've been reprogrammed. I had been resigned to the idea that weight loss was impossible or, at the very least, implausible; that eating clean and living well must be painful and involve sacrifice. I feel like the Love Your Lower Body plan has completely demystified this for me. I've been given the instruction manual for the rest of my life. For the first time in many years, I believe that I am capable of living at a healthy weight. The biggest gift I have ever received is that faith in myself. For that, I am eternally grateful.

Already I've experienced so many huge victories. I'm a singer, and I feel like my voice is stronger thanks to all of this core work. I sleep great and have gained more energy and optimism. Appearance-wise, it has been great watching my body change shape. Places where cellulite used to be are now just solid and lean, and I swear I've lost two chins. I have a long way to go, but that's so fun! It's like I'm being remolded.

I LOVE MY LOWER BODY because:

My tush has completely transformed from what I'd begun to refer to as "Mom buns" (sort of flat and saggy) into a perky, round, firm one. It's like I went back in time 10 years! My legs are stronger and leaner than ever. Boot shopping this fall is going to be fun now that I can fit into tall boots!

Chapter 9

The LOVE Your LOWER BODY Journal

IF I WERE TO ASK YOU TO NAME FROM MEMORY EVERYTHING YOU ATE today, you'd probably be able to list the main meals and snacks that passed your lips. But chances are you would fail to mention—or even remember—that extra snack you had before lunch or the extra dessert after dinner. Our days are so full of activity, and we so often snack mindlessly, that it's easy to forget exactly what we've done.

Keeping track of all of your choices—big and small—in a food and fitness journal can help you stay focused and on track during the Love Your Lower Body program. All of our test panelists kept a log of their daily diet and exercise habits, and many continued journaling after the plan ended. After just a few days of recording their habits, these women realized that seeing their actions on paper kept them accountable. It's easy to understand why: When you must write down all that you eat and do, you automatically put more thought into each bite and each step, skipping snacks you don't need and trying to move more each day. In fact, a study from the Kaiser Permanente Center for Health Research found that people who kept a log of everything they ate lost twice as much weight as those who didn't,[1] and exercise logs appear to have similar effects. In a recent study about effective weight-loss habits, Japanese researchers found that those participants who had successful weight loss over the course of a year were twice as likely to keep a record of their daily habits and were also more likely to record their weight.[2]

I've included space in the following journal for you to record your food and fitness each day. But that's not all. Journals are a great place to chart your likes and dislikes and your progress. You can star your favorite recipes and make note of how you grouped together your workouts each day, commenting on what really worked and what didn't. It may soon become apparent that Chicken Tacos should be on your family's menu each week and that you feel more alert if you do at least 10 minutes of exercise first thing in the morning. These journal pages are the place to record all of the changes you experience on the journey, from how you look to how you feel to the foods you crave. I've given you extra space to write about your mood, your energy level, and any small and large victories you have, such as making it through a full workout without any breaks or fitting into a pair of once-too-tight jeans.

Each week, I provide a question or two to guide your journal writing—but feel free to expand on your own thoughts, too.

I invite you to use these pages to keep yourself committed and to remind yourself of how far you've come. If you recall, I asked you to record your

		BASELINE	
Weight			
Body fat %			
Lean muscle mass			
Chest circumference			
Waist circumference			
Hip circumference			
Right thigh circumference (6" above knee)			
Left thigh circumference (6" above knee)			
Right upper arm circumference (3" above elbow)			
Left upper arm circumference (3" above elbow)			

BEFORE

Paste your photo at baseline here.

AFTER

Paste your photo after completing Week 8 here.

baseline weight and measurements in Chapter 4. You can write those measurements in the table below, then come back every 2 weeks to write in your new measurements. As a reminder, you will need a special scale to record your body fat percentage and other markers, if desired. Otherwise, just make sure you use the same scale for each weigh-in to get an accurate result. To measure the circumference of your waist, hips, legs, and arms, you'll need a tape measure and a friend who is willing to help you. Bending and shifting to hold and read the tape measure on your own can distort your measurements; plus, you want to be sure you measure in the same spots every time.

	WEEK 2	WEEK 4	WEEK 6	WEEK 8

WEEK 1

This week is about easing into the Love Your Lower Body plan because starting a new routine can be stressful. How are you easing into this program so it is less disruptive to your life?

	FOOD (record what you ate)	EXERCISE (record your workouts)	COMMENTS (record your thoughts, moods, energy, accomplishments, etc.)
Day 1:			
Day 2:			
Day 3:			

FOOD	EXERCISE	COMMENTS
(record what you ate)	(record your workouts)	(record your thoughts, moods, energy, accomplishments, etc.)

Day 4:

Day 5:

Day 6:

Day 7:

WEEK 2

Getting on board with this program requires some organization. Take a moment to list the ways you are organizing your life so you eat on plan and get your workouts in.

	FOOD (record what you ate)	EXERCISE (record your workouts)	COMMENTS (record your thoughts, moods, energy, accomplishments, etc.)
Day 1:			
Day 2:			
Day 3:			

FOOD	EXERCISE	COMMENTS
(record what you ate)	(record your workouts)	(record your thoughts, moods, energy, accomplishments, etc.)

Day 4:

Day 5:

Day 6:

Day 7:

WEEK 3

You have a new mat workout this week designed to help you work deeper in your body. Do you notice any changes in your ability to do the exercises?

FOOD (record what you ate)	EXERCISE (record your workouts)	COMMENTS (record your thoughts, moods, energy, accomplishments, etc.)
Day 1:		
Day 2:		
Day 3:		

FOOD (record what you ate)	EXERCISE (record your workouts)	COMMENTS (record your thoughts, moods, energy, accomplishments, etc.)

Day 4:

Day 5:

Day 6:

Day 7:

WEEK 4

You are up and moving all day long with the 10-minute workouts. How is this working for you? Is this easier to do or more challenging? Why?

FOOD (record what you ate)	EXERCISE (record your workouts)	COMMENTS (record your thoughts, moods, energy, accomplishments, etc.)
Day 1:		
Day 2:		
Day 3:		

FOOD	EXERCISE	COMMENTS
(record what you ate)	(record your workouts)	(record your thoughts, moods, energy, accomplishments, etc.)

Day 4:

Day 5:

Day 6:

Day 7:

WEEK 5

How can you make this plan more your own? Have you modified any of the postures to feel better in your body? Have you started experimenting with food, building your own meals based on the Love Your Lower Body guidelines?

FOOD (record what you ate)	EXERCISE (record your workouts)	COMMENTS (record your thoughts, moods, energy, accomplishments, etc.)
Day 1:		
Day 2:		
Day 3:		

FOOD (record what you ate)	EXERCISE (record your workouts)	COMMENTS (record your thoughts, moods, energy, accomplishments, etc.)

Day 4:

Day 5:

Day 6:

Day 7:

WEEK 6

What physical wins have you experienced? Are your clothes fitting more loosely now? Have you noticed tone and definition in places you didn't have it before?

FOOD (record what you ate)	EXERCISE (record your workouts)	COMMENTS (record your thoughts, moods, energy, accomplishments, etc.)
Day 1:		
Day 2:		
Day 3:		

FOOD (record what you ate)	EXERCISE (record your workouts)	COMMENTS (record your thoughts, moods, energy, accomplishments, etc.)

Day 4:

Day 5:

Day 6:

Day 7:

WEEK 7

What have been the biggest changes you've experienced outside of your appearance? Are these workouts affecting the rest of your day?

FOOD (record what you ate)	EXERCISE (record your workouts)	COMMENTS (record your thoughts, moods, energy, accomplishments, etc.)
Day 1:		
Day 2:		
Day 3:		

FOOD (record what you ate)	EXERCISE (record your workouts)	COMMENTS (record your thoughts, moods, energy, accomplishments, etc.)
Day 4:		
Day 5:		
Day 6:		
Day 7:		

WEEK 8

How can you take this program to the next level and make it something that helps you live better beyond these 8 weeks?

FOOD (record what you ate)	EXERCISE (record your workouts)	COMMENTS (record your thoughts, moods, energy, accomplishments, etc.)
Day 1:		
Day 2:		
Day 3:		

FOOD	EXERCISE	COMMENTS
(record what you ate)	(record your workouts)	(record your thoughts, moods, energy, accomplishments, etc.)

Day 4:

Day 5:

Day 6:

Day 7:

Chapter 10

LOVE Your LOWER BODY All Day Long

THE LOVE YOUR LOWER BODY RECIPES BALANCE THE KEY NUTRIENTS required to keep your body and mind in peak condition. Meanwhile, the workouts burn calories and build muscle that will boost your metabolism all day long. But there's more to burning fat than diet and exercise. Part of my job is to give you a deeper awareness of how to live better every moment of the day. As a passionate educator, I'm most excited about your discovering ways to live well *between* the meals and workouts.

It's Not Just About Diet and Exercise

Many factors affect how we look and feel. Studies show that daily stress levels, the amount of time you spend sitting, and how well you sleep at night all influence how your body metabolizes food and stores fat and how happy you feel on a given day. Here are some simple ways to make sure that the hard work you put into this plan really pays off.

Step 1: Move More

Think about how much you move each day. You can count your Love Your Lower Body workouts in this tally, but what I really want you to think about is the activity that goes beyond traditional fitness. Things like walking around the office, carrying laundry up and down the stairs, and even standing on the bus. You may spend dozens of minutes engaged in some kind of gentle physical activity—perhaps even 2 or 3 hours a day—but chances are you spend at least 20 hours of your day not moving much at all.

This inactivity is a big problem, and not just for your waistline: A recent study from England found that too much sitting contributed to a higher likelihood of developing type 2 diabetes and heart disease.[1] In 2011, American Cancer Society researchers found that women who sat more than 6 hours a day were 37 percent more likely to die during a 13-year period than women who sat fewer than 3 hours a day, even if the more sedentary women exercised regularly.[2] In other words, even if you exercise at a vigorous pace for 30 minutes a day, that sweat session won't do you much good if the rest of your day is spent perched in a chair or plopped on a couch.

These are some scary-sounding statistics, but the solution is pretty simple: Spend more time standing, walking, fidgeting, and otherwise moving throughout the day. For years, researchers at the Mayo Clinic have studied how these everyday activities can influence your health, and their findings are incredibly promising. By moving more all day long—standing each time you talk on the phone, walking to and from nearby stores and restaurants, and even washing the dishes by hand rather than loading them in the dishwasher—you'll zap hundreds of extra calories each day, all while helping to regulate your blood sugar, boost your metabolism, and rid your body of fat.

Use these ideas to make every day more active.

• Park a few blocks from your destination so you have to walk a bit more to get there.

• Walk to your coworker's office instead of sending an e-mail.

LET GO OF THE OLD

etting go of old material objects and behaviors is liberating—especially those that don't align with your priorities to find whole-body health. Purge your closets of clothes that don't fit, like the "fat" jeans you hold on to in case you need them. Go through your pantry and donate foods that don't energize you and that sabotage your weight goals. Recycle magazines that make you feel empty and bad about yourself. Stop recording shows that keep you up too late at night. By letting go of old ways, you will have more room in your closet, your pantry, and ultimately your life to live better.

- Get a hands-free headset or use the speakerphone function so you can stand or pace when you're on the phone.

- Tackle your home to-do list: organizing closets, washing windows, and cleaning the floors.

- Ride a bike or walk to errands within a mile of your house.

- Cook with fresh veggies—washing and cutting them will burn calories.

- Schedule walking meetings with coworkers.

- Catch up with friends while strolling through the neighborhood.

- Set a timer on your computer that alerts you to take a break to stretch or walk around every 20 to 60 minutes.

- Limit your tube time. When you watch TV, stand up during commercials, if not during the show.

- Wash your car by hand instead of driving through the car wash.

- Do yard work, such as pruning trees and planting flowers.

One way I add more activity to my day is to *stand* at my computer. I've installed a couple of counter-height desks at our barre3 office so my team and I can move between standing and sitting. At home, I often work while standing at my kitchen counter. It's a small change in habit, but I know that a couple of extra hours spent standing add up! Plus, I've noticed that when I'm standing, I'm more likely to add in other activity, whether that means doing little pliés or walking to refill my water glass or tea mug.

Of course, the 10-minute Love Your Lower Body routines are another way to break up sitting time. Many of the test panelists reported feeling antsy after sitting for too long. They began to crave these short bursts of exercise as a mental break and a way to sustain energy. If I must sit in a chair for long periods of time—if I'm on an airplane or in an important meeting—I figure out ways to keep moving. If you ever spot a woman doing the Love Your Lower Body Standing Stretch in the aisle of an airplane, it might be me!

Step 2: Get Your Z's

What does sleep have to do with weight loss? Plenty! In our time-strapped society, it's easy to think that it's possible—and even harmless—to run on as few as 5 or 6 hours of sleep each night. But resting for anything much shorter than 8 hours can stall weight loss and even cause you to gain: According to a Stanford University study of 1,024 people, those who regu-

CROSS-TRAIN

am a big fan of diversity of movement. I do barre3 so I can do everything else better, from going on brisk walks to taking yoga classes to chasing after my kids. I even pepper in boot camp with my best friends from time to time. You may be surprised to find yourself craving more opportunities to be active. It sounds counterintuitive, but it's true: Once your body gets used to moving more, you might have a hard time sitting still. This happens to a lot of people who begin exercising regularly: You start to seek new ways to move. I observed this among our test panelists. Some added elliptical workouts, while others were inspired to pick up an old sport, like tennis. The Love Your Lower Body workouts didn't make these exercisers tired—they actually jump-started a desire to do even more!

Here's a look at some of the different kinds of exercise you may want to integrate into your life.

MODERATE EXERCISE: Moderate activity is typically defined as any exercise you could do for a continuous stretch of time—that's why it's sometimes also called "endurance training." Your heart rate, breath, and calorie burn increase during moderate activity, but you should still be able to hold a conversation while you exercise. Brisk walking, a jog or bike ride, and fitness classes like water aerobics or yoga fall into this category, and so does a friendly game of tennis or a session on the elliptical machine.

INTERVAL EXERCISE: Intervals are all the rage in the fitness community, and for good reason: Sports scientists have found that short but intense bouts of exercise can provide many of the same benefits of

larly slept 8 hours a night had the lowest BMIs overall.[3] Get fewer than 8 hours of shut-eye and your BMI is likely to rise.

There are a few reasons for this inverse relationship between rest and weight. Subconsciously, when you're tired, your mind starts thinking about ways to get more energy (and a little extra comfort)—which is one reason you may find yourself reaching for candy and other treats after restless nights. This has been documented time and time again. For example, a

more moderate activity in a fraction of the time. During interval exercise, there are typically two basic modes: (1) You are going all out, or (2) you are resting, giving your body a chance to recover from the intense exercise. These types of training are staggered. You might go all out for 20 seconds then recover for 20, repeating this pattern for 5 minutes. On a gym schedule, interval classes might be called "Tabata" (named for a scientist who pioneered some of the interval research) or HIIT (which stands for high-intensity interval training).

STRENGTH TRAINING: More muscle equals a more active metabolism. But sculpted muscles can benefit your body in a number of other ways, including increasing your endurance, reducing your risk of arthritis and osteoporosis, improving your posture, and protecting your body from injuries. The term "strength training" probably brings to mind dumbbells and barbells, but there are lots of other ways to build muscle. Using gym tools like kettlebells and elastic tubing and bands are effective ways to do this. Mind-body classes like yoga and Pilates also count as resistance training, thanks to the amount of effort required from the muscles. Barre3 workouts aren't designed to break down muscle in the same way that intense strength training does, so it's fine to do them day after day. But more rigorous strength-training routines using heavier weights, machines, or other traditional strength-training techniques shouldn't be done back to back, so be sure to take a day's rest between sessions that train the same muscle groups. (For example, be sure to work your biceps every other day, not every day. You can always work your core or your lower body on the opposite days.)

recent study on cravings at the Robert Wood Johnson Medical School in New Jersey found that people who slept fewer than 5 hours a night craved carbs 50 percent more than those who got a more adequate 7 or 8 hours of sleep.

But another reason for this more frequent eating is purely hormonal. When you're sleep deprived, your body produces more ghrelin, the hormone that regulates hunger, and it also makes less leptin, the hormone that tells you when to stop eating. Even if you just polished off a healthy veggie bowl for lunch, that extra ghrelin in your blood will tell your brain that you're still hungry. This hormonal imbalance can cause you to eat extra all day. Continue this sleepless trend for a few days and I can almost guarantee that your waistline will move out, not in.

Also, don't forget about the effect sleep has on exercise. One of the most common reasons I hear from people who skip workouts is that they were too tired to exercise. If you aren't well rested, you may feel fatigued during your workouts, which means you're less likely to push yourself to the place where those quakes and shakes happen. After a workout, proper rest allows your muscles time to relax and recharge. Without it, you may set yourself up for injury, something that can definitely sabotage weight-loss plans.

For some of us, lack of sleep is caused by a scheduling problem—we just aren't allowing ourselves enough time to rest. If this is you, see what changes you can make to turn in early enough to get your 8 hours. According to sleep doctors, the most common environmental causes for a restless night are sleeping in a room that's too warm, too loud, or too bright. If any of these ring true, make the necessary changes to turn your bedroom into a comfortable, quiet, and dark place for rest. My husband and I recently took the TV out of our bedroom. I don't miss it one bit. I am reading again and getting at least 1 extra hour of sleep each night. Be sure to charge your smartphone in a place that's out of reach, as well—it's too tempting to get sucked into that tiny screen every time an update pings, especially when you're trying to get your body into sleep mode.

If you've always had sleep troubles, the changes you've made on this plan toward healthier foods and regular exercise should actually help you get a better night's rest, according to scientific studies.[4] By getting rid of alcohol and coffee, you've eliminated two common causes of sleep problems.

CURB YOUR TV TIME

Looking for more ways to improve your health? The amount of time you spend staring at your television is a major predictor for health problems, and exercise can't counteract the damage. A study from the Harvard School of Public Health found that watching television greatly increases risk of type 2 diabetes, cardiovascular disease, and death from all causes, and other studies report that television time has a direct effect on BMI, with avid television watchers more at risk for obesity.[5] This is bad news for most Americans, who average watching 4-plus hours of television a day, according to the most recent Nielsen report.

The problem isn't the programming. It's the amount of time TV watchers spend glued to the couch. Break up this sitting time and you'll reduce some of the health risks. The next time you watch the tube, stand up and do at least one of your 10-minute workouts. This will break up your sitting time and, according to Brooke Alley, one of our test panelists, may even encourage you to exercise for longer. "When I have the TV on, I often do three workouts in a row without thinking twice," she says.

Skip the hard-to-digest fats and other foods that can lead to tummy troubles and you'll be in even better shape come bedtime. Add moderate exercise to your waking hours and your body will be physically tired by the time you get horizontal. That's why so many doctors prescribe lifestyle change instead of pharmaceuticals for sleep problems—it often is enough.

Step 3: Drink More Water

You know that old wives' tale about drinking more water to speed up weight loss? Well, it works. A recent 12-week study from Virginia Tech found that people who drank 2 cups of water before each meal lost almost 5 pounds more than people who didn't.[6] The researchers are still pinpointing why this happens, but one strongly held theory is that more water in your belly equals less room for food.

Even if you've met your weight-loss goals, it's important to keep your water intake up. Doctors at the Mayo Clinic note that water helps flush toxins from the body's vital organs and carries nutrients to the cells. Adequate water consumption helps optimize digestion, prevent constipation, and can even improve your workouts, according to a study in the *European Journal of Clinical Nutrition*.[7] Drinking enough water can also make your brain work better, improving your mood as well as your memory, according to two separate studies that appeared in the *Journal of the American College of Nutrition*.[8]

So how much H_2O is enough? Surprisingly, that's one thing that researchers haven't wholly agreed on. Water needs can vary by person, climate, and activity level, among other factors, with people who are more active and who live in warmer climates typically needing more water. But there are general guidelines you can use to figure out the right amount for you: For starters, you're likely dehydrated if you regularly feel thirsty or if your urine is anything darker than light yellow.

If you're the measuring type, here are numbers from the Institute of Medicine, the health arm of the National Academy of Sciences: Women should aim to drink around 73 ounces of water a day, or 9 cups. That's a bit more than that other old wives' tale about drinking 8 glasses of water a day, but it's close!

Here's one way I remind myself to stay hydrated: I place four rubber bands on a 12-ounce water bottle. (I bought myself a glass bottle, which doesn't have any sort of aftertaste.) Each time I refill the bottle, I take a band off. I make it a goal to have all of the bands removed by the end of the day. That's 48 ounces of water. When I add up all the other water I get—at meals, in my green tea—I'm drinking more than enough.

Step 4: Minimize Stress

Stress is on the rise, particularly among women. According to the American Psychological Association's 2012 "Stress in America" survey, 43 percent of women say their stress levels have increased in the past year, with a quarter rating their stress levels as an 8 or higher on a 10-point scale.

GIVE YOURSELF PERMISSION

You know how the flight attendant instructs us to first put on our own oxygen mask so that we can then help our children? This same principle applies to exercise and eating right: By making your own health a priority, you'll be better able to take care of others and build meaningful relationships. I've found that if I get up early and get my workout in, I'm able to give more generously to my clients during class. As a parent, when I take care of myself by eating well and getting a good night's sleep, I am much more present with my children, whether playing card games with them or skateboarding. Being good to my body refills my reserves of empathy, energy, and enthusiasm. It makes me able to cope with disappointment, stress, and joy. If you ever begin to feel guilty about putting yourself first, remind yourself that doing so will only help you take care of everyone else in your life.

These women regularly experience fatigue, sleep troubles, headaches, and a lack of motivation as a result of their stress, and they gain weight.

Stress and weight gain are linked in a couple of key ways. Stress triggers your kidneys to release more cortisol, the "stress hormone," which increases appetite and cravings for sugar, according to several studies. In one, published in the journal *Psychoneuroendocrinology,* women consumed more calories and sweets on days they were exposed to stressful situations than on days when their stress levels remained low.[9]

But cortisol also tells the body to hold on to fat during stressful times, which is why even people who follow a healthy diet gain weight when they're stressed. Researchers at the University of California, San Francisco, found that women with the greatest reactions to stress (that is, the women who produced the most cortisol during stressful times) were also the ones who had the most fat in their abdomens, regardless of how fat or thin they were everywhere else.[10] According to researchers at the University of Maryland Medical Center, stress also increases your heart rate and blood

EXERCISE OUTDOORS

Make the most of your workouts by taking your training outside. Whether you do your Love Your Lower Body routines at the park or head out for a morning run around the neighborhood, study after study has found that nature can enhance the benefits of exercise. How can a change of scenery help your health? Exercising outside is more enjoyable than working out inside, according to one British study,[11] and another study—this one from sunny San Diego—found that outdoor exercisers tended to stay active for more minutes than indoor exercisers.[12] Outdoor time can also improve your mood and increase your vitamin D levels, and it may even lower your cortisol levels more effectively than the same workout done indoors.

pressure, speeds up your circulation and your breathing rate, and slows down digestion. For a lot of us, stress can also lead to more tension in our bodies, such as in the shoulders, and to gastrointestinal problems like irritable bowel syndrome. Stress forces the body to function on high alert. This is perfectly okay on occasion, but when stress becomes chronic, it can weaken your immune system and put you at increased risk of heart disease and stroke.

Ready for the silver lining? Exercise is a known way to reduce overall feelings of stress—that's why so many psychologists suggest working out to their anxious patients. Of all the exercises tested for their effectiveness at bringing back feelings of calm, mindfulness-based activities score the highest. Yoga, in particular, is emerging as a proven stress reducer. In one recent study from the Boston University School of Medicine, people either walked or did yoga 3 days a week for 60 minutes. After 12 weeks, the yoga group reported greater increases in mood and less anxiety; they also showed significantly boosted levels of GABA, a neurotransmitter that is associated with feeling good. The walking group also felt better, but not nearly as much.[13]

I often refer to barre3 as "sneaky yoga." Although you won't practice traditional yoga (like chanting "om" or meditating in Savasana), the mindfulness of yoga is very much a part of my barre3 workouts, including this Love Your Lower Body program. The type of small, detailed movements we do requires you to focus inward. If you are focused on your form, alignment, and the small, inner actions of the body, you don't have time to let your mind wander or worry about your life. Instead, you are in the moment, connecting your breath to the movement. This is a meditation of sorts and works wonders to relieve tension. I hope you will find that this mind-body connection sharpens your ability to become more attuned to how other parts of your day trigger stress. This workout travels with you—it truly can help you all day long.

You can harness this power to find calm when you need it. One thing that I do, and that many of the women in the test panel started to do without even being prompted, is to recognize those moments of stress and then interrupt them with a workout. This is how panelist Sarah La Du uses her workouts to help reduce stress: "On most days, right around 3:00 p.m. is when I have trouble focusing on all of the work piling up on my desk. My energy is waning and my anxiety is starting to build. On Week 3 of the program, I realized that interrupting this with a 10-minute workout left me feeling less stressed and better able to focus on a task than before. Plus, I get to check one workout off of my to-do list!"

Michelle Tubbs, another test panelist, found that no matter when she did the workouts, she had an overall sense of calm and well-being that lasted all day, despite her 8 weeks on the plan coinciding with a particularly stressful period: "As the weeks progressed, I was enjoying more and more positive comments about how I looked," said Tubbs. "My extended family kept commenting throughout our family reunion, 'You look great! What are you doing?' Friends I saw regularly were also noticing changes in my body, and they, too, wanted to know 'my secret.' One friend even recently said that my eyes looked much clearer and less fatigued. All of these comments came during an incredibly stressful summer, unlike any other we've had. I think that speaks volumes about the barre3 approach and its positive effects!"

Being aware of your stress levels and your ability to change them is empowering. When I made this connection, I started to make choices that helped me steer clear of a lot of unnecessary anxiety. For example, I began to say no to obligations after 4:00 p.m. so I could sit at the table with my kids for dinner every night. When my business started to take off, I shifted my bedtime up an hour so I could get up with plenty of time to fit in a workout each morning. All of these choices are what ultimately take our results from short-term fixes to long-term whole-body health.

Step 5: Make Healthy Friendships

My mom once told me, "Choose to surround yourself with people who feed you, who make you feel full and happy, rather than people who suck up all the good energy and leave you feeling depleted." It took me some years to fully understand the power of her wise words. Today, I am so thankful for her advice, because encircling myself with people who "feed" me has transformed my life. There was a time when I felt drained because I was taking care of others and not taking care of myself. I was also bombarded with unhealthy choices that challenged my goals to eat well and exercise. Today, I have built relationships with friends, team members, family, and clients who inspire me each and every day to live better. In my experience, surrounding yourself with people who have healthy habits and positive attitudes is contagious. My friends are such a huge influence in my life. My favorite times are when we are exercising together or standing around my kitchen island assembling healthy meals for our kids. My team at barre3 is like an instant injection of positive serum each time I see them—even on my lowest days they elevate me and remind me of my core values. Being aware of how different relationships impact your behavior and how you feel is a big step toward whole-body health.

Raising the Barre

CORI BOYNTON

AGE: 32   POUNDS LOST: 13   INCHES LOST: 7 *including 2 each from her waist and hips*

My weight has always been up and down, but in my early twenties I got to my lowest weight with Atkins. For years, I maintained my weight without any regular exercise. Then my late twenties hit—and along with it, more dates, dinners out, and cocktails. This old plan stopped working. So I began running and the weight slowly came off without any changes to my diet. A few years later, I got into a relationship and it really wrecked my commitment to running. I had a hard time keeping my workouts on a schedule and eating smaller, healthier meals. My boyfriend and I were both gaining weight, and nothing we tried seemed to stop it.

At the first Love Your Lower Body test panel meeting, Sadie described the whole foods approach, which was sort of reminiscent of Atkins—the main change I made was doing more prep work and not relying on fast food. On Sundays, I make a few breakfast and lunch options that I can grab and go—I'd rather eat the same things for 3 days than have to worry about cooking each day.

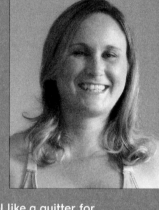

All of my new body fat had made running unbearable—I felt like I was jiggling everywhere—so the controlled barre3 moves were a nice change! I got to stay still and focus on fatiguing my muscles. I love that this way of training doesn't zap my energy in the same way running does. If things started to feel uncomfortable, I would modify the move or just stop for a second. It was great to not feel like a quitter for taking a break—to know that I'm actually going back stronger. I was surprised that doing 10 minutes here and there a few times a day really did wonders. When I didn't want to work out, I would commit to 10 minutes and then see how I felt. Sometimes, that was all I did, but usually it would motivate me to add more exercise. If those first 10 weren't so bad, why not add more? Two weeks in, my boyfriend told me my rear was narrower and more lifted than before.

Within a week of the diet and exercise plan, I noticed my skin was also looking so much better! Not only clearer, but it actually had a glow about it. My diet has improved so much that I no longer have cravings for sugar or bread. In fact, I am amazed how sweet everything tastes now! Some things I used to find irresistible are now unappealing. My energy is up and my posture is better. I feel leaner and sleeker. Almost instantly, my waistline sucked in, which gave me a lot more confidence. It felt better not having my clothes hug me so tight.

I LOVE MY LOWER BODY *because:*

I'm getting stronger. I like seeing new muscle definition and feeling more flexible in my hips. I love the strength of my legs. I especially appreciate them when I want to run fast. They have unlimited potential to carry me to new achievements.

Chapter 11

LOVE Your LOWER BODY for Life

WE ALL HAVE DIFFERENT MEASURES OF SUCCESS. FOR ONE OF THE TEST panelists, success meant buying—and wearing—her first pair of skinny jeans. For another, it meant changing her tastes so much that she craved kale chips, not potato chips. My measure of success was retention: All 27 women who started the Love Your Lower Body test panel also finished it. These women didn't just *last* 8 weeks on this plan, they *thrived*. They told me that the ease of the 10-minute workouts toned and shaped their bodies better than any other programs they'd tried. The nutrition component inspired them to cook more at home—and to create recipes made up of whole foods for whole-body health. They came in with specific weight-loss goals, and this program delivered. But what they gained was even more powerful: They learned how to make exercise and eating well a way of life and something that felt very much their own.

At the end of the 8-week Love Your Lower Body test panel, these women were transformed. One had lost 18 pounds, and another had dropped nearly 12 inches. But the most monumental changes were the little ones, the ones that were hard for other people to see but that affected these women far more than the numbers on a tape measure or scale. Annie Eeds, a client of mine who has lost more than 75 pounds (and counting!) on this plan, coined a phrase for these successes that I just love: "nonscale victories."

Nonscale victories were overflowing by the end of the 8 weeks: Jennifer Dashney-Longbine had an easier time keeping up with her twin toddlers. Michelle Tubbs kept her cool during an incredibly stressful summer. Jessica Klein had enough energy to take her small business to the next level. Frayn Masters's painful sciatica disappeared. Zoe Murillo made healthy meals her whole family would eat. Carie Behe started to sleep through the night, getting an uninterrupted 8 hours. Sarah La Du's posture improved. Alex Nowlin cured her sweet tooth. I could go on and on. All of these women signed up for Love Your Lower Body to get shapelier legs and a more lifted tush, and they all succeeded. However, they'll be the first to tell you that they also got so much more. I hope you see yourself in some of these success stories. Weight loss is a wonderful goal, but it really is these other victories that make big change worthwhile.

Next Steps

Being healthy is a constant practice. It isn't something that happens all at once. It's something we chip away at. Although our official 8 weeks together are over, it doesn't mean you need to put this plan aside. There is probably at least one healthy habit—and quite possibly more—that you've adopted along the way that will stay with you for good.

I know from experience that self-improvement can be daunting. It can be especially difficult to give up old behaviors and attitudes that have become deeply ingrained in who you are and how you live. Transitioning to a healthier lifestyle isn't something you can do in just one or two steps. It requires that you remake your everyday activities, from how you grocery shop to how you spend your leisure time. I have been on this journey for years now, and I'm happy to report that it gets better and easier as you go.

My hope is that the past 8 weeks have been illuminating and rewarding for you, that you had an easier time transitioning to eating whole foods than you expected, and that the workouts actually felt good and made you feel even better after. Be proud of your successes big and small. Each workout you did, each healthy meal you made, was a step in the right direction. Some of these healthy habits will stick and others won't. If you don't live this way all year long, I suggest you repeat this program once or twice a year. That way, at least one new healthy behavior will stay with you each time. Eventually, as your healthy habits grow, being on the program and off it won't feel all that different. These positive lifestyle changes will gradually seem less disruptive and become easier and easier to adopt. Before you know it, you won't even be on or off the plan—you'll just be living in a healthier, more mindful, and more balanced way.

Measuring Your Success

There are two different ways to measure how this plan worked for you: on-scale victories and non-scale victories. You may have kept track of both of these, or you may have opted to focus on one. Either way, it's important to measure your success and take into account how far you've come.

On-scale victories are straightforward. You simply look back at your initial measurements and see how you compare now. A weight loss of 1 to 2 pounds a week is safe, and studies show this rate often leads to lasting weight loss. Changes in inches and pounds will be individual and pretty noticeable; as fat disappears, muscle moves in, creating a leaner physique. You'll also notice how your pants hang on your waist differently and how you fit into smaller sizes when you go shopping for a new outfit. These are changes that can be precisely measured.

Off-scale victories are much more ambiguous, and, really, anything goes. Below is a list of common successes I've heard people talk about in my studios and on the test panel. You may have experienced some of these and others of your own. As you read through this list, take a few moments to think about—and even write down—some of your successes big and small.

- Measuring taller with improved posture

- Holding plank for a full minute

- Being able to balance better (during workouts and all day)

- Skipping second helpings at mealtime

- Sleeping more soundly

- Shaving your legs more easily

- Ditching your unhealthy afternoon snack habit

- Being complimented on how much younger/fitter/happier you look

- Experiencing improvements in flexibility

- Craving healthy foods

- Forgetting what that "afternoon slump" feels like

- Walking up the stairs without getting winded

- Feeling sexy again

- Braving a new exercise class

Keep on Going

If you'd like to keep living the Love Your Lower Body way or are revisiting this routine and ready to come back, here are some tips for continued results.

- Use the Portion Prescription (page 46). This visual guide to the specific percentages of protein, healthy fat, and fiber you want on your plate can help take the guesswork and measuring out of food prep. Photocopy it and tape it to your fridge. By simply "eyeballing" your plate, you'll make having a healthy meal even easier.

- Try your own recipes. Blending the old and the new can make the plan feel familiar and exciting all at once. Use my nutrition formula to update old favorites and to create your own recipes from scratch.

- Mix and match workouts. The 10-minute workouts are designed to balance the various muscle groups. Feel free to do them in any order you like to craft new programs each week that will keep you motivated and excited about exercise.

- Get deeper. In Chapters 5 and 6, I share some tricks for getting deeper into the postures. Glance back at those occasionally to make sure you are pushing your body to its limits.

- Start your mornings with the 10 Transformative Minutes. By doing this foundation routine each and every morning, you get at least 10 minutes of exercise in every day—and you get it done before life has a chance to get in the way.

- Set nutrition rules. Making exceptions to your diet can snowball, so decide ahead of time what parts of the program you are committed to and what tenets you will be more flexible about. Maybe you plan on drinking wine on special occasions, or you really want one cup of coffee each morning. Pick a plan and stick with it.

There's a whole spectrum of ways to transition from these 8 weeks of Love Your Lower Body. Here's how some of the women on the test panel chose to move on after the plan.

Jennifer Dashney-Longbine decided that she was ready to keep going with the workout and diet.

I'm all in. I've realized that I can't "sort of" do this. I have to do this all the way. I feel like I can see the light at the end of the tunnel—that I'm finally on my way to reaching my goal weight. It's so much easier to look at this as a lifestyle now that I already have 8 weeks under my belt—and now that my belt is smaller! Now that the cravings are gone and I'm in the habit of working out, I don't have any desire to stop. I don't feel like I'm on a diet anymore. This is just how I live.

Brooke Alley still eats mostly whole foods and does the 10-minute workouts.

I'm following about 65 to 70 percent of the plan. Some changes are going to be for the long haul, like eating whole foods such as whole grain brown rice instead of instant white rice, and using whole dairy instead of reduced fat. I really avoid sugar now, and I have habituated to eating protein with fat and fiber to stabilize my blood sugar. I did add a little alcohol back in, but it's pretty minimal—a glass of wine or two a week. However, other things never stuck. I still drink a cup of coffee a day, but I drink less coffee overall and have added in green tea with no sweetener almost every day. I will continue the workouts and the morning 10 Transformative Minutes as often as possible—I like how they make me feel.

Sarah La Du takes breaks on holidays and special occasions.

I decided to take a week off for my birthday to see how I felt. But my "off" week still had 4 days of working out, and my meals were mostly Love Your Lower Body–approved, just because that's what's in my kitchen and what sounds good. I indulged in cake, a lemon tart, and some cocktails this week, but I also ate salads and salmon. I didn't lose any weight during those 7 days, but I didn't gain any, either. I was willing to sacrifice progress to spoil myself a little over my birthday week, and I'm still happy to have done that. Having a start and end date for my "vacation" week was pivotal. It let me feel good about my decision and not worry about backsliding or going back to my old ways. At the end of the week, I was excited to get back to the plan. Now that I'm officially off the program, I know I'm making healthier choices because I want to, not because I'm supposed to.

Carie Behe is practicing moderation.

On other diets, I would restrict myself for certain periods of time to the extreme, so much so that when something disrupted that strict routine, like a work trip, I would fall off the wagon in a major way. On Love Your Lower Body, I haven't restricted myself to that point, and that has been helpful. So while I'm being good this week eating whole foods and smaller portions, I know that next week, when my dad comes to visit, it will be okay to allow myself to indulge, eating a few dinners out or drinking beer or wine. I've truly learned that moderation is the key with this, and that it is okay to indulge once in a while. I've never had that strategy in the past.

Zoe Murillo is following a looser version of the plan.

I never gave up my morning espresso, although now I enjoy it with whole milk and maple syrup. I eat almost no sugar and have cut way back on bread. I'm trying to include fiber, fat, and protein in most meals and snacks, and I try to move more all day. I make new recipes with ingredients mostly off of the shopping list and have barre3-approved sweets on hand for my sugar cravings. I've actually tried to bring back some of my old behaviors—like eating frozen yogurt or drinking a little wine—but they no longer taste good to me.

Jessica Klein is still committed to the workouts:

I am in 100 percent with the exercise and I would say 92 percent with the diet. When I do my 10 minutes, I'm not dripping in sweat, but it's strengthening the places I need and doing wonders for my stress management. When I start to move, that tightness in my chest literally disappears. I recently got back from a short family vacation, and I've had some dinners out and a glass of wine here or there, but I don't enjoy it as much. I think my taste buds have changed, for the better. When I've had a sugary treat or alcohol, it really doesn't make me feel good. At the beginning of this program, the sugar, alcohol, and caffeine were the major modifications, since I was already gluten and dairy free. When I went back to my old way of eating, I noticed my energy levels went down and my sleep wasn't as good. So I'm back. I'm so glad we had the first 8 weeks to establish a baseline and see how awesome I could feel without these things in my diet. This way, when social events come up and old habits or cravings kick in, I have something to weigh my choices against.

April Abernethy relaxes a little on the weekends.

I have a minimum-adaptation rule for the changes I've made. Some of this is also based on past experience and how quickly things can get away from you if you don't plan. So I have to do three of the longer barre3 workouts each week, and then I fit in as many 10 minutes as I can in between. I try to follow the eating plan a minimum of 5 days a week and then my own modified plan at least 2 days a week because I want the flexibility to not build guilt in around food. I have added coffee back in, but I limit it to 1 cup a day with just coconut milk for creamer.

Taking the Long View

When I first kicked off the Love Your Lower Body test panel, I wanted to give our panelists a glimpse of what they could look and feel like if they turned the next 8 weeks into a permanent daily practice. I decided to invite two women who changed their lives by living the barre3 way. Robyn Conley Downs and Annie Eeds exemplify what my formula of small changes in exercise and diet can do over a period of months and years. Little did I know that by inviting these women to give a pep talk, I would be recruiting two of the most amazing health coaches around. Throughout the 8-week program, they not only followed the plan alongside the testers, they also provided wisdom, support, guidance, and motivation. I was so inspired by Robyn and Annie's dedication, transformation, and overwhelming positivity that I wanted to share their stories with you, too. Here's a look at what repeating this program can do and how letting the habits build and grow over time can transform you—inside and out—for good.

Annie Eeds

Has lost more than 75 pounds with barre3

In college I gained and lost the same 30 or 40 pounds, and in the 5 years after graduating, I gained another 50. I remember the moment I decided to lose weight like it was yesterday. It was fall of 2011, and I had just been diagnosed with insulin resistance (the stage right before type 2 diabetes) and polycystic ovarian syndrome. My friends were talking about how they couldn't imagine weighing over 200 pounds, except maybe when they were pregnant. When I got home, I got on the scale. It said 220 pounds—and I definitely wasn't pregnant.

So I scheduled my first barre3 class at the Vancouver, Washington, studio. It was daunting. I was more than 70 pounds overweight, and I had major shakes and quakes during most of the exercises. But the studio was welcoming, and once I got over my insecurities, I took a second class, and a third, and a fourth.

After about 6 months of exercise, I wanted to shift my eating habits, too. I signed up for a 4-week barre3 food and fitness challenge. It was a big change from the processed foods I normally ate. I tried new veggies and learned how much food I needed to feel satisfied and energized. The DIY bowls and salads are now a staple in my home, and the meals I make follow the Portion Prescription. During those 4 weeks, I lost 7 pounds and 3 inches—and that was just the beginning.

Over time, this way of living has only gotten easier. Each week, I plan meals, shop, and prep food to make my life smoother. Sure, I have to be "picky" when ordering at restaurants, but to me it's worth getting what I pay for. I practice in the studio several times a week, and I do a 10-minute online workout each morning before my shower. I eat really well 90 percent of the time. When I choose to splurge, I make sure it's worth it! After 18 months living the barre3 lifestyle, I have lost 78 pounds. I weigh less than I did in high school, and I have never been so fit!

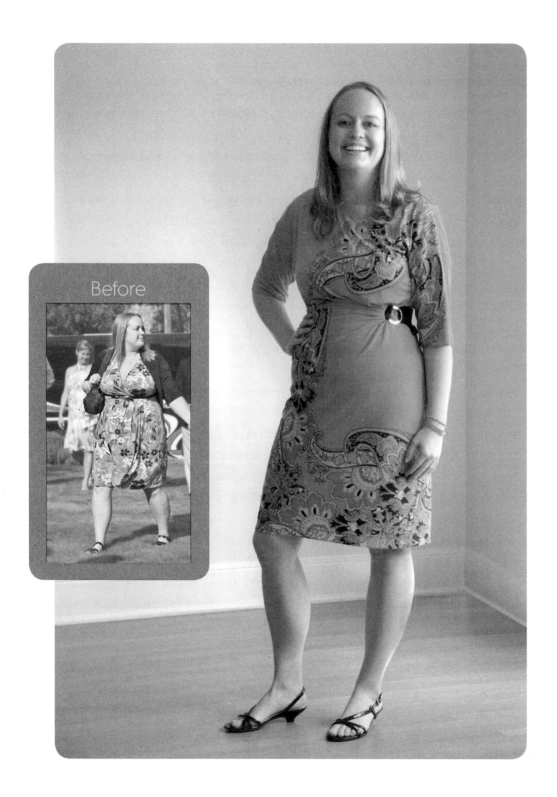

Before

Robyn Conley Downs

Has lost more than 40 pounds with barre3

In high school, I was an extremely dedicated athlete who spent a minimum of 3 hours a day playing basketball. But in the decade following school, work, stress, and life crept in and extra pounds crept on. When I first heard about barre3, it sounded like a means to an end—the end, of course, being to lose weight. It was late fall of 2012, and in the 8 months since my daughter was born, I had tried, valiantly and unsuccessfully, to get my weight down. (I was carrying an extra 20 pounds when I got pregnant, and a difficult pregnancy caused me to gain an additional 60.) For several months, I tried running, counting calories, and counting points. I was starving, frustrated, and, worst of all, not losing any weight. I could manage everything else in my life successfully—being a full-time student while working 60-plus hours a week and being a mom and wife—but my weight felt like something out of my control.

When I started consistently doing barre3 workouts and following the diet, I knew the program was different. The workouts were extremely challenging, but they made me feel strong and centered instead of drained and exhausted. I loved that I could do barre3 online workouts while my daughter napped or during breaks between work and school. I committed to the eating plan and felt nourished and satisfied. I fully embraced eating fiber, fat, and protein at every meal. I gave up sugar and alcohol, something I had thought I would never be willing to do. After a few weeks, I was amazed to find my cravings were gone, my energy was up, and my body was changing.

Barre3 has allowed me to connect back to my younger, fitter self. I remember this revelation clicking in one of my favorite instructor's classes, during a ridiculously hard legwork sequence. There I was, quads burning, breathing hard, sweat literally dripping off my forehead, and I had this profound moment where I realized that I could be an athlete again. I had thought I was too old, too mom-ish, too far from who I used to be, but at that moment, I realized I was wrong. Today, I look a lot more like the fit athlete I was in my teens. I'm so happy when I look in the mirror and my reflection matches the image of myself I've always had in my mind.

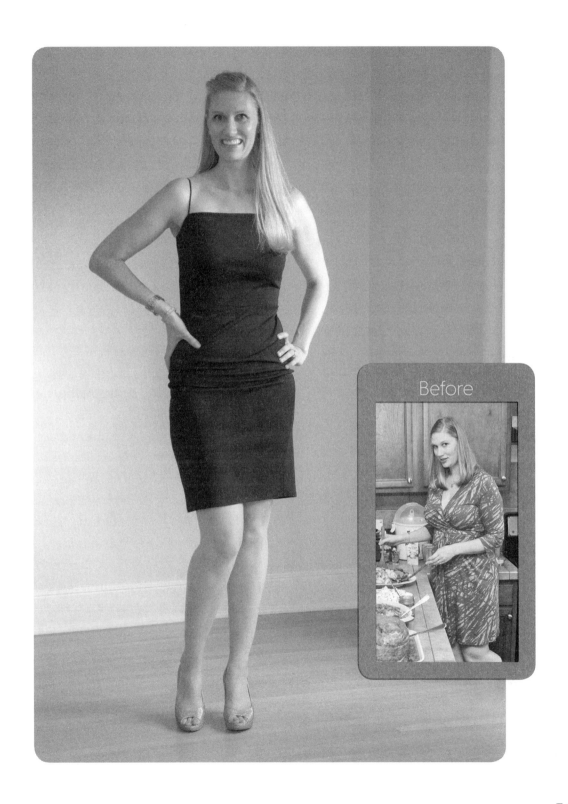

Before

Raising the Barre

MEGAN SCHENDEL

AGE: 30   POUNDS LOST: 13.8   INCHES LOST: 9¼ *including 2½ from her waist and 1½ from her hips*

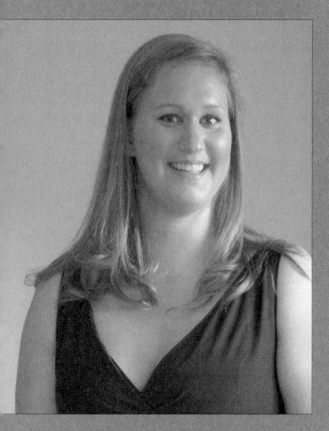

I was a Division 1 college athlete and have had a very strong and capable body for the majority of my life. But all of that changed when my husband and I decided to start a family. Five years ago, during my first pregnancy, I gained about 35 pounds. I stayed active throughout my pregnancy, but the weight did not come off easily. After I weaned my daughter at 12 months, I was able to drop the weight briefly, but within a month of reaching my goal weight, I became pregnant with my son. Even though I stayed just as active, if not more so, the second time around I gained over 50 pounds. I held on to 30 of those pounds through two failed attempts at Weight Watchers, weaning my son at 18 months, and several diets, including a low-carb plan.

When I applied for the Love Your Lower Body test panel, my emotions were mixed: I was hopeful that it would work and also fearful that I might fail once more. Luckily, I got into the groove right away with the eating plan. I had virtually no cravings. I wasn't even tempted by sugar, which has always been my drug of choice. I felt frustrated at the occasional social event, but not because I really wanted to eat the pizza, chips, and ice cream. I was simply dismayed to not have enough, or sometimes any, healthy options to fuel my body.

The exercise, too, felt natural right from the start. I really liked how the plan allowed me to integrate exercises into my life: Ten-minute segments are perfect for my busy life as a stay-at-home mom. That's pretty much the amount of time I can sneak in before my kids make it impossible to continue. I learned to squeeze in 10 minutes while cooking dinner, when I was at the park with my kids, or when the kids were welcoming daddy home. I also love that I don't need to be in workout clothes and doubled-up sports bras for support. I learned that I can achieve a great workout whenever I happen to have a few minutes. It was so freeing to not have to completely structure my day around exercise; I structured my exercise around my life!

For me, weight loss was a definite success, but I was also amazed at how out of touch I was with my core. I saw such a difference in my waist on this program. Shorts I needed to be 10 pounds lighter to wear now fit because I've tightened my core so much and because I've gotten rid of my belly bloat. I've also experienced a drastic drop in stress eating and bingeing, which have plagued me since adolescence. I feel so much stronger and steadier than I did before. Simple things like squatting down to get something out of a bottom cabinet are so much easier than before.

I LOVE MY LOWER BODY *because:*

My legs haven't looked this good since I was a Division 1 volleyball player. They are so toned and sleek, and my butt is lifted. People have asked what I'm doing and if I'm a runner since my legs look so great. Nope! It's LYLB!

Endnotes

INTRODUCTION

1. A. Romero-Corral et al., "Normal weight obesity: a risk factor for cardiometabolic dysregulation and cardiovascular mortality," *European Heart Journal* 2010 Mar; 31(6): 737–46, doi:10.1093/eurheartj/ehp487.

CHAPTER 1

1. A. C. King et al., "Behavioral impacts of sequentially versus simultaneously delivered dietary plus physical activity interventions: the CALM trial," *Annals of Behavioral Medicine* 2013 Oct; 46(2): 157–68, doi:10.1007/s12160-013-9501-y.

CHAPTER 2

1. R. K. Dishman, "Compliance/adherence in health-related exercise," *Health Psychology* 1982; 1(3): 237–67, doi:10.1037/0278-6133.1.3.237.

2. W. H. Ettinger Jr. et al., "A randomized trial comparing aerobic exercise and resistance exercise with a health education program in older adults with knee osteoarthritis: the Fitness Arthritis and Seniors Trial (FAST)," *Journal of the American Medical Association* 1997; 277(1): 25–31, doi:10.1001/jama.1997.03540250033028.

3. F. Tsofliou et al., "Moderate physical activity permits acute coupling between serum leptin and appetite-satiety measures in obese women," *International Journal of Obesity and Related Metabolic Disorders* 2003 Nov; 27(11): 1332–39.

4. C. R. Salas, K. Minakata, and W. L. Kelemen, "Walking before study enhances free recall but not judgement-of-learning magnitude," *Journal of Cognitive Psychology* 2011; 23(4): 507–13, doi:10.1080/20445911.2011.532207.

5. T. Nabetani and M. Tokunaga, "The effect of short-term (10- and 15-min) running at self-selected intensity on mood alteration," *Journal of Physiological Anthropology and Applied Human Science* 2001 Jul; 20(4): 231–39.

6. C. Manohar et al., "The effect of walking on postprandial glycemic excursion in patients with type 1 diabetes and healthy people," *Diabetes Care* 2012 Dec; 35(12): 2493–99, doi:10.2337/dc11-2381.

7. T. S. Church et al., "Effects of different doses of physical activity on cardiorespiratory fitness among sedentary, overweight or obese postmenopausal women with elevated blood pressure: a randomized controlled trial," *Journal of the American Medical Association* 2007 May 16; 297(19): 2081–91.

8. A. B. Sullivan, E. Covington, and J. Scheman, "Immediate benefits of a brief 10-minute exercise protocol in a chronic pain population: a pilot study," *Pain Medicine* 2010 Apr; 11(4): 524–29, doi:10.1111/j.1526-4637.2009.00789.x.

9. S. C. Moore et al., "Leisure time physical activity of moderate to vigorous intensity and mortality: a large pooled cohort analysis," *PLoS Medicine* 2012; 9(11): e1001335, doi:10.1371/journal.pmed.1001335.

CHAPTER 3

1. G. A. Bray, S. J. Nielsen, and B. M. Popkin, "Consumption of high-fructose corn syrup in beverages may play a role in the epidemic of obesity," *American Journal of Clinical Nutrition* 2004 Apr; 79(4): 537–43.

2. M. Garaulet et al., "Timing of food intake predicts weight loss effectiveness," *International Journal of Obesity* (Lond) 2013 Apr; 37(4): 604–11.

3. K. Maruyama et al., "The joint impact on being overweight of self reported behaviours of eating quickly and eating until full: cross sectional survey," *British Medical Journal* 2008 Oct 21; 337: a2002, doi:10.1136/bmj.a2002.

4. A. J. Oliveira-Maia, S. A. Simon, and M. A. L. Nicolelis, "Neural ensemble recordings from central gustatory-reward pathways in awake and behaving animals," *Methods for Neural Ensemble Recordings* (Frontiers in Neuroscience), 2nd ed., Miguel A. L. Nicolelis (Boca Raton, FL: CRC Press, 2008).

5. M. R. Lowe and M. L. Butryn, "Hedonic hunger: a new dimension of appetite?," *Physiology & Behavior* 2007 Jul; 91(4): 432–39.

CHAPTER 4

1. E. E. A. Cohen et al., "Rowers' high: behavioural synchrony is correlated with elevated pain thresholds," *Biology Letters* 2010 Feb 23; 6(1): 106–8, doi:10.1098/rsbl.2009.0670.

2. J. F. Hollis et al., "Weight loss during the intensive intervention phase of the weight-loss maintenance trial," *American Journal of Preventive Medicine* 2008 Aug; 35(2): 118–126, doi:10.1016/j.amepre.2008.04.013.

CHAPTER 9

1. J. F. Hollis et al., "Weight loss during the intensive intervention phase of the weight-loss maintenance trial," *American Journal of Preventive Medicine* 2008 Aug; 35(2): 118–26, doi:10.1016/j.amepre.2008.04.013.

2. M. Nakade et al., "What behaviors are important for successful weight maintenance?" *Journal of Obesity* 2012; 2012: 1–7, doi:10.1155/2012/202037.

CHAPTER 10

1. E. G. Wilmot et al., "Sedentary time in adults and the association with diabetes, cardiovascular disease and death: systematic review and meta-analysis," *Diabetologia* 2012; 55(11): 2895, doi:10.1007/s00125-012-2677-z.

2. A. V. Patel et al., "Leisure time spent sitting in relation to total mortality in a prospective cohort of US adults," *American Journal of Epidemiology* 2010 Aug 15; 172(4): 419–29, doi: 10.1093/aje/kwq155.

3. S. Taheri et al., "Short sleep duration is associated with reduced leptin, elevated ghrelin, and increased body mass index," *PLoS Medicine* 2004 Dec; 1(3): e62, doi:10.1371/journal.pmed.0010062.

4. A. C. King et al., "Moderate-intensity exercise and self-rated quality of sleep in older adults: a randomized controlled trial," *Journal of the American Medical Association* 1997 Jan 1; 277(1): 32–37.

5. A. Grøntved and F. B. Hu, "Television viewing and risk of type 2 diabetes, cardiovascular disease, and all-cause mortality: a meta-analysis," *Journal of the American Medical Association* 2011 Jun 15; 305(23): 2448–55, doi:10.1001/jama.2011.812.

6. E. A. Dennis et al., "Water consumption increases weight loss during a hypocaloric diet intervention in middle-aged and older adults," *Obesity* 2010 Feb; 18(2): 300-7, doi:10.1038/oby.2009.235.

7. R. J. Maughan, "Impact of mild dehydration on wellness and on exercise performance," *European Journal of Clinical Nutrition* 2003; 57: S19–23.

8. A. Adah, "Cognitive performance and dehydration," *Journal of the American College of Nutrition* 2012 Apr 1; 31: 71–78.

9. E. Epel et al., "Stress may add bite to appetite in women: a laboratory study of stress-induced cortisol and eating behavior," *Psychoneuroendocrinology* 2001; 26: 37–49.

10. E. S. Epel et al., "Stress and body shape: stress-induced cortisol secretion is consistently greater among women with central fat," *Psychosomatic Medicine* 2000 Sep–Oct; 62(5): 623–32.

11. C. J. Thompson et al., "Does participating in physical activity in outdoor natural environments have a greater effect on physical and mental wellbeing than physical activity indoors? A systematic review," *Environmental Science and Technology* 2011 Mar 1; 45(5): 1761–72, doi:10.1021/es102947t.

12. J. Kerr et al., "Outdoor physical activity and self rated health in older adults living in two regions of the U.S.," *International Journal of Behavioral Nutrition and Physical Activity* 2012 Jul 30; 9:89, doi:10.1186/1479-5868-9-89.

13. C. C. Streeter et al., "Effects of yoga versus walking on mood, anxiety, and brain GABA levels: a randomized controlled MRS study," *Journal of Alternative and Complementary Medicine* 2010 Nov; 16(11): 1145–52, doi:10.1089/acm.2010.0007.

Index

Boldface page references indicate photographs. <u>Underscored</u> references indicate boxed text.

M

V

Vegetables

W

Walnuts

Water